T0323870

THE PSYCHOLOGY OF MENOPAUSE

What physical and psychological changes can I expect when going through menopause? How can I protect my well-being during menopause? How can I ensure a good menopause experience?

The Psychology of Menopause provides a useful and positive guide to understanding the psychological, social, and sexual changes that occur during and following menopause. Going beyond hot flushes and HRT, it focuses on how to enhance psychological well-being by looking at the science behind women's lived experiences of perimenopause and postmenopause. The book explores key psychological issues during this transition, such as the risk factors associated with mood and anxiety, the changing social and personal roles for women in midlife, the impact on relationships, and the reasons for brain fog.

By putting women's psychological well-being at the heart of this stage of life, *The Psychology of Menopause* provides a much-needed examination of the psychological, social, cultural, and interpersonal aspects of the transition into and beyond menopause.

Marie Percival is an academic, author, practitioner, and researcher. With over 18 years of experience teaching psychology and psychological therapies to undergraduate and postgraduate students at higher educational institutions in the United Kingdom and Ireland and dealing with countless clients during this period, she has acquired extensive knowledge in this field.

THE PSYCHOLOGY OF EVERYTHING

People are fascinated by psychology, and what makes humans tick. Why do we think and behave the way we do? We've all met armchair psychologists claiming to have the answers, and people that ask if psychologists can tell what they're thinking. The Psychology of Everything is a series of books which debunk the popular myths and pseudo-science surrounding some of life's biggest questions.

The series explores the hidden psychological factors that drive us, from our subconscious desires and aversions to our natural social instincts. Absorbing, informative, and always intriguing, each book is written by an expert in the field, examining how research-based knowledge compares with popular wisdom, and showing how psychology can truly enrich our understanding of modern life.

Applying a psychological lens to an array of topics and contemporary concerns – from sex, to fashion, to conspiracy theories – The Psychology of Everything will make you look at everything in a new way.

Titles in the series:

For more information about this series, please visit: www.routledge textbooks.com/textbooks/thepsychologyofeverything/

THE
PSYCHOLOGY
OF MENOPAUSE

MARIE PERCIVAL

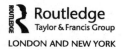

Routledge
Taylor & Francis Group

LONDON AND NEW YORK

First published 2025
by Routledge
4 Park Square, Milton Park, Abingdon, Oxon OX14 4RN

and by Routledge
605 Third Avenue, New York, NY 10158

Routledge is an imprint of the Taylor & Francis Group, an informa business

British Library Cataloguing-in-Publication Data
A catalogue record for this book is available from the British Library

ISBN: 978-1-032-57213-0 (hbk)
ISBN: 978-1-032-57212-3 (pbk)
ISBN: 978-1-003-43834-2 (ebk)

DOI: 10.4324/9781003438342

Typeset in Joanna
by Apex CoVantage, LLC

To my precious daughter Claire, I dedicate this book to you with all my love.

May this book offer you support and guidance as you move through life, and may it serve as a reminder of the love and admiration I hold for you.

You are, and will forever remain, the most wonderful gift I could ever hope for.

CONTENTS

PREFACE

Welcome to *The Psychology of Menopause*.

There has been a significant increase in discussions surrounding menopause in recent times, indicating that it is no longer a taboo topic. The extensive coverage of menopause in the media, academia, and health sector is welcome news.

Social media platforms are flooded with menopause support groups that connect women worldwide, allowing them to share their experiences, provide support during distressing moments, or simply offer a listening ear on difficult days. This is undoubtedly a step in the right direction. It is heartening to witness such progress, especially considering the dark past when menopause was shrouded in stigma and secrecy and associated with insanity and negative stereotypes.

However, menopause remains a complex topic, with polarised views on its meaning and management. Consequently, there is an abundance of conflicting information available, which can be confusing and anxiety-inducing for both those currently experiencing menopause and younger women who will go through it in the future. It is crucial to navigate through this sea of information with caution.

Advancements in the field of medicine, specifically hormone replacement therapy (HRT), have had a profound impact on the lives of women going through menopause. This is particularly true for those experiencing severe and frequent vasomotor symptoms, such as hot flushes and night sweats. HRT has also been found to have a protective effect against other chronic conditions that may arise during the post-menopausal stage of life.

However, it is important to acknowledge that women's experiences with menopause symptoms can vary greatly. There is no one-size-fits-all approach when it comes to treating these symptoms. It is evident that relying solely on a biological model to address menopause often falls short of comprehensive menopause care. The range of symptoms associated with menopause is vast and constantly expanding. Therefore, a more comprehensive approach is needed to manage and alleviate these symptoms effectively.

I advocate for a broad perspective on menopause, one that acknowledges its biological aspect as common sense. Menopause is a natural occurrence for women fortunate enough to live long enough to reach this stage of life. However, menopause does not exist in isolation. There are other issues, situations, and life events that coincide with this phase, making it essential to extend the conversation to include the psychological and social factors associated with this inevitable biological event.

The aim of this book is to provide a concise, evidence-based summary of the extensive body of academic literature and research on menopause and to extend the conversation beyond the polarising debate of medicalisation of menopause versus viewing menopause as a natural event. Instead, I advocate for recognising the psychological and social factors that both contribute to, and are consequences of menopause. In other words, I offer a biopsychosocial approach to menopause experience.

This book is intended for anyone interested in women's health and well-being, regardless of their menopausal status, whether you are a woman approaching menopause, already in the post-menopausal stage, a partner, friend, employer, or someone working in healthcare supporting women during menopause, this book is designed for you. The writing style is informal and conversational, designed to be easily understood and accessible to all readers.

I choose to use the term "woman" and "women" in this discussion, although I acknowledge that individuals with a uterus can encompass a diverse range of gender identities, including non-binary, trans men, and other gender populations.

I invite you to consider a holistic approach to understanding and managing menopause. I welcome your thoughts and views on issues presented in this book. Please visit my website, www.psychologyofmenopause.com, where you can contact me and access additional information and insightful blog posts about various aspects of menopause. I welcome your feedback.

Best wishes,

Marie Percival

1

MENOPAUSE THROUGH THE AGES

INTRODUCTION

The main objective of this chapter is to provide a detailed summary of the menopause experience and not to simply list menopause symptoms. We will explore how menopause is understood and experienced across different cultures and throughout history, shedding light on the societal and medical perspectives surrounding this transformative phase in a woman's life. We will also discuss global initiatives that aim to raise awareness about menopause, showcasing the advancements made to educate and support women during this transitional period. Additionally, we will provide valuable guidance on how to navigate menopause in the workplace, addressing the unique challenges and considerations that middle-aged and older women may face. By combining evidence-based information, historical insights, cross-cultural perspectives, and practical guidance, this chapter aims to provide a holistic understanding of the meaning and management of menopause and will serve as a valuable resource for medical and allied health professionals and all individuals seeking knowledge to support women at this transformative stage of their lives.

DOI: 10.4324/9781003438342-1

MENOPAUSE DEFINED

Menopause is a natural biological process that marks the end of a woman's menstrual cycles and her ability to get pregnant. It is a normal part of the ageing process, and it happens at about the age of 51 for women in Europe, Britain, and the United States. This age can vary by ethnicity, but the research is mixed. To diagnose menopause correctly, your doctor will take a detailed medical history and give you a physical examination.

Everyone with a menstrual cycle will go through menopause during their lifetime if they are fortunate enough to live that long. By 2030, it is estimated that 1.2 billion women will be menopausal worldwide, with 47 million entering menopause each year. Menopause is one of many life stages for women and marks the end of their reproductive years. After this, women typically cannot conceive unless they undergo specialised fertility treatments, though such cases are rare. The majority of women experience menopause between the ages of 45 and 55, which occurs due to the cessation of ovarian follicular activity and a decrease in oestrogen levels.[1]

If you have not had a menstrual period for 12 consecutive months and there is no other apparent reason or medical intervention, you have entered natural menopause. It is possible for some women to experience menopause at an earlier age, even before reaching 40. This early onset, known as "premature menopause," can be attributed to various factors such as chromosomal abnormalities, autoimmune disorders, or unidentified causes. Menopause can also occur earlier than age 51 due to surgery or medical treatment such as a hysterectomy. Unfortunately, we just can't predict when an individual woman will experience menopause, although there are associations between the age at menopause and certain demographic, health, and genetic factors.

Menopause is divided into three stages:

Perimenopause: This is the stage before menopause and can start several years before the actual onset of menopause. During perimenopause, oestrogen levels fluctuate, leading to irregular menstrual cycles and various symptoms such as hot flushes, night sweats, mood changes, and disturbed sleep. This happens because oestrogen levels are declining and can last from a few months to several years. Around half of all women notice physical and/or emotional symptoms during this time.

Menopause: Menopause proper is officially defined as the point when a woman has not had a menstrual period for 12 consecutive months.

Postmenopausal: Post menopause is the stage after menopause when hormone fluctuations tend to stabilise, and many of the symptoms experienced during perimenopause diminish. However, some women may continue to experience symptoms such as vaginal dryness and changes in bone density.

CHANGES ASSOCIATED WITH MENOPAUSE

While not classified as a disease or condition, menopause is accompanied by various symptoms. The hormonal shifts during this period can impact a person's physical, emotional, mental, and social well-being. However, the severity and type of symptoms experienced during and after menopause vary greatly from individual to individual. While some may only experience minimal symptoms or none at all, others may face severe symptoms that significantly impact their daily activities and overall quality of life. Unfortunately, some women endure these symptoms for several years.[2]

There are well over 40 recognised symptoms associated with menopause, but it is unlikely that any one woman will have all of them. They include:

- Hot flushes and night sweats. Hot flushes are a sudden feeling of heat in the face, neck, and chest, often accompanied by flushing of the skin, sweating, palpitations, and acute feelings of physical discomfort that can last several minutes.
- Changes in the regularity and flow of the menstrual cycle, culminating in menstruation stopping altogether.

- Vaginal dryness, pain during sexual intercourse, and incontinence.
- Difficulty sleeping/insomnia.
- Changes in mood, depression, and/or anxiety irritability.
- Difficulties in concentration, being able to focus, and memory.

Menopause profoundly impacts women's health, impacting body composition, metabolism, weight, and cardiovascular risk. While women initially have a cardiovascular advantage over men, this diminishes as oestrogen levels decline postmenopause. The transition can weaken pelvic support structures, elevating the risk of pelvic organ prolapse. Simultaneously, bone density loss significantly contributes to increased rates of osteoporosis and fractures. These changes underscore the critical need for comprehensive healthcare and support for women during this transformative life stage.

Unsurprisingly, hot flushes and night sweats (excessive perspiration) in bed at night are challenging, and apart from disturbing sleep, these vasomotor symptoms also have a negative impact on women's mental health and overall well-being and quality of life. Menopause symptoms are usually confined to the perimenopausal period; however, they can occasionally persist past the final period and into the postmenopausal stage.

It is important to note that while all women will experience hormonal changes during the menopausal transition, not all have vasomotor symptoms.[3] While population estimates vary, it is thought that over 70% to 80% of all women experience hot flushes at some point during this time. As we've seen, menopause has a significant impact on different aspects of a woman's life, such as sleep, mood, and cognitive function. This means that hot flushes, night sweats, and sleep quality are important issues that can have specific implications for both physical and mental health. Research has shown that there are several key risk factors affecting these symptoms, including the level of education, smoking, and low mood. It is worth noting that obesity, previously believed to protect you during the perimenopausal and early postmenopausal stages, is actually now considered a risk factor for experiencing these symptoms.[4]

CONTEMPORARY TREATMENTS

When it comes to considering treatment for menopausal symptoms, there's no one-size-fits-all remedy. It needs careful and thoughtful consideration, as well as discussions with your healthcare provider. Fortunately, you have several treatment options available to you for managing the symptoms. The most important first step is to talk to your doctor, taking into account the frequency and severity of your symptoms, as well as the impact they have on your quality of life, both physically and mentally. Your doctor will evaluate your needs and medical history and talk you through the treatment they think will be most likely to benefit you. These options include lifestyle changes, HRT, complementary and alternative therapies, and psychological therapy. Let's look at each of them.

HRT

The history of HRT is filled with controversy, making it unwise to label it definitively as either safe or unsafe. It's important to remember that HRT is a form of treatment, and when it comes to managing our health, we must carefully consider the risks and benefits of undergoing any treatment.

The impact of HRT varies depending on the specific hormones used (oestrogen, progesterone, or testosterone), whether they are administered individually or in combination, the method of administration (such as pills, patches, or gels), and the timing of initiation (whether it is started near menopause or later). There is substantial evidence that HRT, particularly oestrogen, can be beneficial for menopausal symptoms, especially for hot flushes. Many women have experienced significant improvements in their lives due to HRT. While the ongoing debate regarding the advantages and disadvantages of HRT is expected to continue, ultimately, the decision of whether the benefits of undergoing HRT outweigh the risks remains a personal choice (with your doctor's advice).

The media often sensationalises the debate surrounding hormone replacement therapy (HRT), portraying it as either helpful or harmful. However, it is important to recognise that this narrow and divisive perspective overlooks the substantial advancements made in understanding HRT. Rather than regarding conflicting scientific opinions with scepticism, it would be more useful to view them as vital for the progression of knowledge.

ALTERNATIVE THERAPIES

Some women choose not to undergo HRT but prefer to explore complementary and alternative interventions, which offer a wide range of options. These treatments can be categorised into three main groups:

Mind-body: Mind-body practices encompass a range of techniques that can have a profound impact on overall well-being. These practices include hypnosis, relaxation exercises, biofeedback training, meditation, and the use of aromatherapy. By engaging both the mind and body, these practices aim to promote a sense of balance and harmony.

Natural health products: There is a wide variety of products that are derived from nature and offer potential benefits. These natural products include herbs, vitamins, minerals, and dietary supplements. They are often used as complementary or alternative approaches to traditional medicine, with the goal of supporting optimal health and wellness.

Alternative or complementary medicine: Alternative medicine encompasses various traditional healing practices that originate from different cultures and traditions. These practices, such as traditional Chinese medicine, reflexology, acupuncture, and homeopathy, have been used for centuries to address a wide range of health concerns. Although they may differ in their philosophies and techniques, they share a common focus on holistic well-being and the belief in the body's innate ability to heal itself.

A 2019 review conducted by Johnson and colleagues[5] found mixed results regarding the effectiveness of natural products, and there were even some safety concerns associated with certain interventions. The review indicated that mind-body practices, such as hypnosis and relaxation techniques, may help reduce stress and alleviate some menopausal symptoms. Specifically, hypnosis was consistently shown to be effective in reducing hot flushes. At the moment, there is not enough evidence to support the use of natural products in alleviating menopausal symptoms, and it is important to exercise caution when considering any treatment, traditional, complementary, or alternative medicine.

LIFESTYLE

Of course, adopting a healthy lifestyle at any stage of life is beneficial. It makes sense that healthy choices can alleviate the temporary symptoms of menopause, and this is fully supported by research. HRT is not suitable for everyone, and for those women who are taking HRT but still experiencing menopausal symptoms, managing their lifestyle can also be effective. Incorporating regular exercise and maintaining a balanced diet, with an emphasis on consuming more vegetables, fruits, fibre-rich foods, and fish while reducing meat intake, may help. Exercise has been proven to enhance mood, improve heart health, and potentially alleviate hot flushes. Studies have shown that women who smoke tend to experience more severe hot flushes, which is yet another reason to quit. Also, stress-relieving practices such as yoga, deep breathing exercises, and massage therapy can help a lot. As we've seen, managing stress levels and getting enough high-quality sleep are crucial for overall physical and mental well-being. In Chapter 7, we will provide ten key exercises, with a focus on psychology and behavioural changes that can assist with physical and mental well-being and brain health during the menopausal transition and postmenopause. These exercises can help you establish positive health habits that can easily be integrated into your daily routine.

PSYCHOLOGICAL THERAPIES

Symptoms such as low mood, anxiety, or sleep difficulties are common among women during the perimenopause stage, and for some women, they may wish to focus on talk therapy or psychological interventions to cope with their symptoms. Research has shown that counselling and psychotherapy are helpful for people with all types of different issues, dealing with life in general, from low self-esteem, relationship issues, depression, anxiety, to workplace stress – all the things that can complicate and disrupt our lives from time to time. But these therapies are especially helpful for women in midlife. The challenge is it is difficult to know what the symptoms are attributed to fluctuating hormones during menopause or if the feelings of low mood, anxiety, irritability, forgetfulness, and general malaise are a result of other life stressors that coincide with this stage of life. Things like adult children leaving home, caring for elderly parents, dealing with relationship issues, divorce or death of a loved one, awareness of one's own mortality, change in social roles, or changes in employment or career can all have profound effects. Counselling and psychotherapy can provide a safe, non-judgemental space to discuss these issues and also give you time to reflect on life choices and space to re-evaluate your values and goals in life.[6]

Cognitive behavioural therapy (CBT) is a widely used evidence-based psychological intervention known for its effectiveness in addressing various menopausal symptoms, such as hot flushes, depression, and anxiety.[7] CBT is a time-limited approach that focuses on modifying thoughts and behaviour to alleviate symptoms. It may involve psychoeducational components, motivational interviewing, and other evidence-based strategies to improve quality of life during this stage of life. The North American Menopausal Society recommends CBT for reducing the distress associated with vasomotor symptoms, although it is not specifically recommended for addressing their frequency.[8] In November 2023, the National Institute of Clinical Excellence (NICE) included CBT as a potential treatment for menopause symptoms in their draft guidelines. This recommendation acknowledges that menopause is a multifaceted experience, and what may work for one person may not work for another. While HRT can be highly effective, some women may find that combining HRT with CBT provides significant relief from their menopause symptoms. This update represents a significant advancement, providing women with more options and flexibility in managing their menopause.

HISTORICAL BELIEFS AND ATTITUDES

Has our understanding of menopause changed throughout history? Let's explore some strange beliefs and attitudes surrounding this phase in a woman's life.

We first heard of the word menopause, which is attributed to a French doctor, Chales-Pierre-Louis de Gardanne, in 1821. The concept was not original to him – it was described about 100 years earlier, but there was no name for it. In the 1700s, doctors began to write about a condition they described as "the cessation of the periodical discharge, in the decline of life, and the disorders arising from that critical change of constitution." In other words, they wrote about a syndrome of symptoms and problems affecting one gender – women – at a specific time in life.[9]

Several doctors in the same era describe women reporting episodes of flushing and sweating that sound like what we call today hot flushes (in the United States, they are more commonly called hot flashes).

The mid-18th century witnessed the emergence of the first widely read advice literature on menopause, featuring titles like "Advice to Women of Forty Years." Throughout the 19th century, medical professionals made groundbreaking discoveries about the nervous system, leading to a greater understanding of the causes of various disorders, including those associated with menopause. Consequently, behavioural symptoms began to take centre stage in discussions surrounding menopause. One notable figure during this time was Edward Tilt, who authored the first comprehensive book on menopause in English titled "Change of Life in Health and Disease." Tilt's work, particularly his second edition published in 1857, speculated that menopause could potentially contribute to alcoholism, mania, and even provoke violent tendencies in women, with potentially fatal consequences.[10]

Tilt was one of the pioneering physicians who quantified the symptoms he witnessed in his patients. The most prevalent symptoms reported were hot flushes, bleeding, nervous irritability, various types of pain, and what he referred to as pseudo-narcotism – a state of cognitive vegetative functioning. According to his perspective, menopause represented a crucial period characterised by heightened nervous irritability, rendering women's health vulnerable. However, once this stage was passed, women could anticipate many years of good health.

Despite the changing attitudes and treatments over time, menopause continues to be an inescapable reality. It is not a matter of choice. This natural and significant life event affects half of the population, yet why is it often associated with fear and apprehension? The historical, social, cultural, and medical factors surrounding menopause have shaped our current perceptions and understanding of this stage in a woman's life.

In ancient times, menopause was surrounded by mystery and misunderstandings. Various cultures had different beliefs about menopause, ranging from associating it with wisdom and renewal to considering women going through menopause as becoming insane. The ancient Greeks, for instance, saw menopause as a natural process where women acquired wisdom and transformed into wise elders. Likewise, Asian societies celebrated menopause as a significant phase in a woman's life, marking a transition and a new beginning. In numerous societies throughout the Middle Ages, menopause was associated with negative beliefs and ideas. It became intertwined with superstitions, witchcraft, and even demonic possession. Women going through menopause were frequently shunned, labelled as witches, and subjected to various forms of prejudice because of the physical and emotional changes they experienced. The lack of knowledge and understanding surrounding menopause greatly contributed to the stigmatisation and marginalisation of women during this natural stage of life.[11]

As far back as 1563, a Venetian physician named Giovannie Marinello believed that menopause was the cause of various health problems affecting different parts of the body. According to Marinello, if women were no longer able to bear children, they would suffer from a lack of purpose and would experience a decline in their overall well-being.

> Those (women) in whom they (periods) have stopped or do not come: like those whom they are to end for reasons of age, are always infirm and most of all in those parts of the body which are connected to and have some kind of correspondence with the uterus, such as the stomach and the head; thus as soon as the periods stop, pain arises, eye disorders, weak sight, vomiting, fever . . . the disorderly uterus rises or descends all the time or commits other actions difficult to endure. From this soon a tightness of the chest arises, faintings of the heart, breathlessness, hiccups and other troublesome accidents, from which the woman sometimes dies.

Colombat de L'Isere, in a chapter on the change of life in 1845, stated that "compelled to yield to the power of time, women now cease to exist for the species, and henceforward live only for themselves." He went on: "She now resembles a dethroned queen, or rather a goddess whose adorers no longer frequent her shrine. Should she still retain a few courtiers, she can only attract them by the charm of her wit and the force of her talents."[12]

Charles Meigis, in a letter to his class in 1848 entitled Change of Life, asked,

> What does she expect save grey hairs, wrinkles, the gradual decay of these physical and personal attractions, which heretofore have commanded the flattering image of society? The pearls of the

mouth become tarnished, the hay-like odour of the breath is gone, the rose has vanished from her cheek.

The female body has almost exclusively been defined by male doctors. Overwhelmingly, their attitudes have been mired in negative, demeaning, and undisguised disgust. American gynaecologist Dr. Robert Wilson, author of the best-selling 1966 Feminine Forever book, declared that they were all "castrates."[13]

How many strange taboos and myths still surround menopause? As a stage of life and as a female experience, the topic has, until recently, remained in darkness, not to be discussed. Unfortunately, some outdated ideas about this time in a woman's life have managed to survive. In David Rueben's 1969 bestseller book Everything You Always Wanted to Know About Sex but Were Afraid to Ask, Reuben described the woman at the mercy of her decreasing hormone production:

> When a woman sees her womanly attributes disappearing before her eyes, she is bound to get a little depressed and irritable. Having outlived her ovaries, they may have outlived their usefulness as human beings. The remaining years may be marking time until they follow their glands into oblivion.

(p. 365)

Despite the disrespectful and demeaning attitudes towards women experiencing menopause, significant progress has been made in treating its symptoms. However, the use of HRT has sparked intense debate and controversy in the past, which still persists today.

TREATMENTS

Treating the symptoms of menopause has certainly changed a lot over the years. Thankfully, the days of using opium, extracting oestrogen from the urine of pregnant women and horses, and relying on remedies like Lydia Pinkham's vegetable tonic or the Change-O-Life elixir are all long behind us. Other treatments included cupping, cold water therapy, and even clitoridectomy (the surgical removal of the clitoris).

In the modern age, as medical science progressed and our understanding of the female reproductive system deepened, menopause started to become a topic of medical interest. It was in the late 19th century that the term 'menopause' was first coined, establishing it as a distinct medical condition. This led to the development of various treatments aimed at alleviating the discomfort and symptoms associated with this stage of life.[14]

Let's fast forward to the 20th century, a time when it was discovered that equine oestrogen could be used as a hormone treatment for menopause symptoms. In 1942, the very first oestrogen product was introduced to the market under the name Premarin. Interestingly, advertisements during the 1950s were not only targeted at women but also aimed at men. Thanks to the immense popularity of Dr. Robert Wilson's bestselling book, Feminine Forever, the sales of HRT skyrocketed in the years following its release. Advertisements for Premarin touted it as a solution for menopause, promising to preserve a woman's youth and beauty. These hormone pills promised to make women "pleasant to live with once more."[15]

From the 1940s until the 1970s, women were prescribed oestrogen for menopause. However, in 1975, it became apparent that taking oestrogen without another hormone called progestogen, known as 'unopposed' oestrogen therapy, increased the risk of endometrial cancer. As a result, the sales of Premarin plummeted. It wasn't until the addition of a progestogen to a lower dose of oestrogen was discovered to mitigate this risk that sales picked up again. This combination therapy, marketed as Prempro, gained popularity.[16]

The resurgence in sales of HRT was further fuelled by aggressive marketing and the portrayal of menopause as a debilitating condition that required treatment. By the early 1990s, Premarin became one of the most widely prescribed drugs in the United States.[17]

The initial decades of HRT use provided evidence supporting its effectiveness not only in alleviating menopausal symptoms but also as a preventive treatment for certain chronic conditions, including bone health and heart issues. In fact, in 1988, it received approval from the US Food and Drug Administration as a preventative treatment for osteoporosis. Additionally, evidence was emerging that suggested that HRT could potentially benefit heart disease prevention. As a result, a large-scale study was initiated in 1991 that would significantly alter the course of HRT.[18]

In the 1990s, the Women's Health Initiative (WHI) trial was a groundbreaking study that had a significant impact, but unfortunately, not in a positive way. According to endocrinologist Megan Ogilvie, it was one of the most detrimental events for women's health in a long time. It did a disservice to an entire generation of women and possibly even two generations.[19]

The primary objective of the WHI was to investigate the effects of HRT, along with other interventions, on the leading causes of death and disability in postmenopausal women. The study aimed to examine the incidence of cancer, cardiovascular disease, and osteoporosis. It is crucial to note that the focus was not on testing the effectiveness of HRT for alleviating menopausal symptoms.

Alarmingly, in 2002, the research was abruptly halted. During the initial phase of the trial, researchers made some concerning observations. They found that women with a uterus who were taking combined HRT experienced a higher risk of developing coronary heart disease and breast cancer. However, there were also some positive findings: a decrease in osteoporotic fractures and colorectal cancer.

Ultimately, the study found that the risks associated with HRT outweighed the potential benefits, leading to the discontinuation of the trial. The media frenzy surrounding this news was immense, causing women to become anxious about the headlines. As a result, many of them decided to discard their medication, and doctors became hesitant to prescribe HRT. This sudden shift in behaviour left pharmaceutical companies in a state of panic, as they faced the possibility of legal action and lawsuits from patients. Consequently, funding for HRT and research in women's health began to dwindle.[20]

The repercussions of the Women's Health Initiative (WHI) study were far-reaching. Not only did doctors stop prescribing HRT, but they also ceased to receive education on menopause. The training for medical professionals no longer included information on menopause, and financial support for HRT products decreased.[21]

Interestingly, in 2017, Professor Robert Langer revealed that the results of the WHI study had been misreported. Some of the researchers involved were shocked to discover that the trial had been prematurely terminated. This revelation shed new light on the study and raised questions about the negativity surrounding the publication of the results.

Unfortunately, the lack of education on menopause remains a problem for both trainee and practicing doctors. Unless they actively seek out knowledge or have a specific interest in the subject, their understanding of menopause is limited. However, from 2019, there have been government initiatives worldwide that aim to address this issue by placing a greater emphasis on women's health during midlife. But not every woman sees menopause as something that needs treating medically, and for that reason, it is important to acknowledge cultural differences in the meaning and management of menopause.

CULTURAL VARIATIONS

Western women have a wide range of perspectives when it comes to menopause. It's not surprising that their views and attitudes towards this stage of life are very much influenced by their own experiences of symptoms – in particular, their frequency and intensity. For some women, menopause can be a challenging and negative experience, negatively impacting their quality of life and leading to feelings of depression, anxiety, and difficulties in relationships. On the other hand, there are women who view the end of their reproductive years as inconsequential and experience little to no symptoms.

It is important to understand that each woman's own experience and interpretation of menopause is unique, and It's not my intention to generalise or stereotype any particular culture. However, cultural attitudes and beliefs surrounding menopause, as well as lifestyle factors and socio-economic status, do have an influence on women's experiences.

Interestingly, when comparing different ethnic groups, we can see some interesting differences in their experiences of menopause. While it is crucial to recognise the variations within and across cultures, research tells us that:[22]

- Menopause and its associated symptoms are often heavily medicalised in Western societies. However, traditional Chinese medicine takes a different approach, viewing menopause (also known as juejing) as a natural part of the ageing process, and the symptoms can be managed through the use of balancing foods and herbs.
- In Japan, there is no direct translation for the term 'hot flush,' and menopause is referred to as 'konenki,' which conveys ideas of energy, rejuvenation, and renewal. In Japanese culture, this stage of life is seen as a time of transition and new purpose rather than being associated with loss and fear.
- Ayurveda is a natural system of medicine that originated in India more than 3,000 years ago. It sees menopause not as a disease but as a period of transition. It is considered a crucial time in a woman's life when she has the opportunity to prioritise her health and well-being in all aspects – physically, mentally, spiritually, and sexually.
- In contrast, Mayan women from Mexico often have negative attitudes towards menstruation and pregnancy. As a result, menopause is viewed as a time of greater freedom and is eagerly anticipated.

We know from research that attitudes and beliefs towards menopause, along with lifestyle factors and socio-economic status, can influence women's experiences. Despite these differences, one thing remains clear: menopause is a significant phase in a woman's life that can have a profound impact on her physical and emotional well-being and her personal and professional life. In recent years, governments worldwide have made remarkable strides in raising awareness about menopause and its impact on women's lives in the workplace.

MENOPAUSE IN THE WORKPLACE

As mentioned previously, every woman's menopause experience is different, from those who have mild, infrequent symptoms to those that are deeply distressing and disruptive in their lives. Some women have a completely neutral experience. We have also learned that for years, women were expected to soldier on, doing their best to conceal the physical and mental manifestations of the so-called change, not to mention the difficulties with impaired cognitive function or brain fog.

Research carried out in Ireland by The Menopause Hub[23] found that 45% of women say that they feel their menopause symptoms have a negative impact on their work and 47% of women needed to take a day off work due to their symptoms and don't feel comfortable telling their employer the reason why.

In Ireland, it is estimated that approximately 600,000 women are currently experiencing perimenopause or menopause. It seems that employers are finally becoming aware of the necessity to offer appropriate support for this significant portion of the workforce.[24]

Experiencing a hot flush can be quite challenging to hide, leading to discomfort and embarrassment, especially when surrounded by others in a workplace or a shared workspace. Cognitive problems such as difficulty finding words and experiencing brain fog are also common symptoms that many women encounter during menopause. Furthermore, mood swings and anxiety are prevalent among perimenopausal women. In addition to these challenges, disrupted sleep caused by night sweats can make it difficult to maintain focus and concentration. Therefore, it is crucial to explore effective strategies for managing menopause while at work. This can be achieved by examining various government initiatives that aim to support women during this phase of their lives.

In the UK, a staggering 13 million women face perimenopause or menopause, representing one-third of the female population. An overwhelming 80% experience noticeable symptoms, significantly impacting their work performance and participation. A study by the

Chartered Institute of Personnel and Development reveals a troubling statistic: two-thirds of working women aged from 40 to 60 years who have experienced menopausal symptoms report a predominantly negative impact on their professional lives. These findings underscore the urgent need for workplace policies and societal changes to support women during this critical life stage.

Of those who were negatively affected at work:

- 79% said they were less able to concentrate.
- 68% said they experienced more stress.
- Nearly half (49%) said they felt less patient with clients and colleagues.
- 46% felt less physically able to carry out work tasks.

Further research by the Fawcett Society found that one in ten women surveyed who were employed during menopause left work due to menopause symptoms.

MENOPAUSE AS A DISABILITY?

In February, 2024 the Equality and Human Rights Commission (EHRC) published new workplace guidance to help employers understand their legal obligations in relation to supporting women with long-term symptoms that have a substantial impact on how a woman may carry out her normal work duties. In this regard, the symptoms could be considered a disability, and as such, a woman is protected under disability discrimination law.

In the UK, the Menopause Task Force has introduced guidance for employers, made reasonable adjustments, such as proper ventilation and flexible working hours, and encouraged a culture of speaking about menopause to all staff and for menopausal women to feel that they can have a conversation about their symptoms with their line manager.

Furthermore, it is essential for employers to recognise the possibility that certain employees may be going through a challenging menopause transition. As a result, they should provide support, such as offering paid time off to attend medical appointments. In some cases, larger organisations arrange for wellness speakers to discuss various health topics, including menopause. This not only benefits female employees but also allows male and younger female employees to gain insight into the experiences of their colleagues.

Education and training programmes for line managers and supervisors, as well as fostering a culture of open communication about menopause and women's health during midlife, along with practical support measures in the workplace and the implementation of well-being initiatives, all contribute to a promising start. Until recently, menopause was not widely discussed in the workplace, but there is still ample room for improvement, even with the progress that has been made. Historically, there has been a sense of shame or embarrassment surrounding the symptoms of menopause. In fact, menopause, particularly hot flushes, has often become the subject of jokes or light-hearted remarks, referred to as a "tropical moment." Additionally, there has been a lack of understanding and awareness regarding the common symptoms. While many may associate hot flushes with menopause, they may be completely unaware that anxiety, fatigue, memory loss, and depression are also prevalent symptoms that can significantly impact a woman's daily life and her ability to perform at her fullest potential in the workplace.

Menopause is not solely a concern for women; it is a matter that affects society as a whole. Although there have been encouraging advancements made by employers in addressing this issue, there is still much work to be done. We have indeed made significant progress in recent years, but it is crucial that employers adopt a comprehensive and inclusive approach.

Establishing comprehensive awareness and support resources is crucial in every workplace. Women should feel empowered to request accommodations without shame, perform their duties in a secure environment, and engage in open dialogues with colleagues and supervisors to foster an inclusive culture. Essential support measures should include robust sick leave policies and accessible medical and psychological support. It is imperative that women feel confident addressing their symptoms, while managers receive proper education on supporting them through these transitions. This approach ensures a workplace that respects and accommodates women's health needs, promoting equality, and productivity.

CONCLUSION

We have learnt in this chapter that menopause is a significant milestone in a woman's life, and while some women experience it without any issues, others face a range of physical, psychological, and cognitive symptoms. Menopause is a complex journey that unfolds in stages, from perimenopause to postmenopause, each bringing unique physical and emotional shifts. The most common are vasomotor symptoms such as hot flushes, night sweats, and chills, but research has shown that the frequency and severity of these symptoms vary greatly among women going through the menopause transition. Throughout history, cultures have viewed and handled menopause differently, shaping women's experiences through varied societal attitudes. Some societies respect it as a transition to wisdom, while others stigmatise or view it solely as a medical issue. In workplaces, menopause remains a critical yet often ignored issue, impacting women's well-being and work performance. It's crucial to address menopause through supportive policies, so that women are sure to manage this phase with respect and minimal disruption. By promoting understanding and open conversations about all aspects of menopause, we can better support women through this life stage, both in their personal and professional lives.

NOTES

1 Newson (2019).
2 Talaulikar (2022).
3 McCall and Potter (2022).
4 Avis et al. (2018).

5   Johnson et al. (2019).
6   Percival (2023).
7   Mann et al. (2012).
8   Hunter (2020).
9   Bezzant (2022).
10 Foxcroft (2010).
11 Mattern (2021).
12 Bezzant (2022).
13 Wilson (1966).
14 Bezzant (2022).
15 Bezzant (2022).
16 Bezzant (2022).
17 Bezzant (2022).
18 Bezzant (2022).
19 Bezzant (2022).
20 Bezzant (2022).
21 Bezzant (2022).
22 Bezzant (2022).
23 Dignam (2021).
24 Dignam (2021).

2

UNDERSTANDING AND MANAGING MENOPAUSE – HOW CAN PSYCHOLOGY HELP?

INTRODUCTION

The journey towards achieving optimal health is multifaceted, and healthcare experts are well aware of this fact. Over the past five decades, health psychologists have recognised the profound influence that psychological and social factors have on both our physical and mental well-being. They also acknowledge that experiencing physical or mental health issues can give rise to additional psychological and social challenges. This realisation is encouraging because it means that the field of psychology is well-equipped to explore and address the complexities surrounding menopause.

Despite advancements in medical treatments for menopause related symptoms, it is equally important to acknowledge that a holistic approach that takes into account psychological and social factors is essential for a comprehensive understanding of menopause. By incorporating these aspects into their practice, healthcare professionals can develop more effective strategies to support women during and after this transitional phase of life.

DOI: 10.4324/9781003438342-2

In this chapter, we will explore the ways in which health professionals can navigate the intricacies of menopause, with a focus on incorporating psychological and social considerations. By doing so, we aim to provide a comprehensive understanding of how menopause impacts women's health and well-being. Through this exploration, we hope to challenge societal norms and advocate for a more compassionate and holistic approach to menopause care.

HEALTH AND WELLNESS

By 2030, there will be an estimated population of 1.2 billion menopausal and postmenopausal women worldwide, with 47 million new entrants each year.[1] To effectively address the current global trend of raising awareness and providing treatments for menopause, we need a conceptual framework that explains its complexities. But what kind of model should this be? Should a model of menopause include psychological factors such as thoughts, emotions, and behaviours, or social factors like the availability of support, stress, and interpersonal relationships? Is a model that solely focuses on the biological aspects of menopause enough? Or do we need additional concepts to fully understand the intricacies of menopause during midlife and older age? Before we address these questions, let's explore the characteristics of biomedical and biopsychosocial perspectives on health.

BIOMEDICAL VERSUS BIOPSYCHOSOCIAL MODEL OF HEALTH AND ILLNESS

The biopsychosocial model of health and the biomedical model represent contrasting approaches to understanding and addressing health and illness. The biomedical model focusses primarily on biological and physical factors in explaining and treating disease, emphasising the role of genetics, pathogens, and physiological processes. In contrast, the biopsychosocial model, introduced by George Engel in 1977, considers the interconnected influence of biological, psychological, and social factors on an individual's health and well-being.[2]

In the biomedical model, diseases are often viewed as resulting from specific biological and physiological abnormalities, such as infections and genetic predisposition. Treatment approaches typically revolve around targeting these underlying biological mechanisms through medication, surgeries, or other inventions aimed at directly treating the pathophysiology of the disease. Medical practitioners acknowledge the psychological and social factors as consequences of illness or symptoms, for example, hot flushes and night sweats in menopause may result in low mood, but traditionally, they have failed to consider the role of psychosocial factors as contributing factors to menopause symptoms.[3]

THE MEDICALISATION OF MENOPAUSE

Despite the ongoing discussion surrounding the excessive medicalisation of menopause in mainstream media and academia, it would be unwise to dismiss the valuable knowledge gained from medical advancements, specifically hormone replacement therapy. The importance of embracing these insights cannot be overstated, as they have the potential to greatly improve women's health and well-being during this significant life stage. While it is crucial to examine the influence of medicalisation on women's experiences critically, we must not discount the benefits that arise from scientific progress in this field.

Menopause, a natural biological process in a woman's life, has historically been stigmatised and misunderstood. However, the availability of hormone replacement therapy (HRT) has brought about significant positive changes for women facing the challenges of menopause. By replenishing declining hormone levels, HRT can alleviate various symptoms such as hot flushes, night sweats, vaginal dryness, and mood swings. It has also been shown to reduce the risk of osteoporosis and cardiovascular diseases, which are prevalent concerns for postmenopausal women.[4]

Critics argue that the medicalisation of menopause (making it a disease) perpetuates societal pressures on women to conform to unrealistic standards of youth and beauty. They claim that by pathologising a natural process, women are led to believe that menopause is a problem that needs fixing. While these concerns should not be dismissed lightly, it is important to recognise that medical advancements have provided women with options and support during a time that can be challenging both physically and emotionally.[5]

We need to strike a balance between acknowledging the medicalisation of menopause and appreciating the benefits it brings. It is imperative that healthcare providers and society as a whole offer comprehensive support, education, and resources to empower women in navigating this significant life stage. That said, relying solely on a biomedical approach to manage menopause is inadequate, given the myriad of symptoms and complexities of menopause at this stage of life. By exploring the psychological and social aspects of menopause, health psychologists can shed light on various issues that women may face during this time. This includes addressing concerns such as mood fluctuations, sleep disturbances, changes in body image, and challenges in interpersonal relationships. By examining these factors through a psychological lens, we gain a deeper understanding of how they contribute to the overall well-being of women experiencing menopause. Recognising the potential of hormone replacement therapy and other non-medical interventions, women can make informed decisions about their health and well-being during and after this transitional phase.

LIFESTYLE MEDICINE

As we celebrate the increasing life expectancy (refer to Chapter 6 for further details), the desire to live longer in good health is a commendable goal. However, the question arises: is it achievable? By embracing the wealth of research on how our lifestyle choices impact our health and well-being, we can potentially look forward to a longer and healthier life filled with vitality, energy, and fewer instances of illness-related disabilities. These principles are equally relevant when considering menopause. It is commonly known that women experience more symptoms during the perimenopause phase. However, it is important to recognise that some women may continue to experience symptoms during the early stages of postmenopause. Even when menopause symptoms subside, the ageing process continues, presenting new challenges and potential health issues. By understanding the impact of our lifestyle choices on our overall well-being, we can strive for a longer and healthier life.

Lifestyle medicine is an evidence-based approach that recognises lifestyle as a leading cause of disease and, therefore, as an appropriate medical intervention alongside usual medical care. Although the practice of lifestyle medicine has been around for thousands of years, it has only come to prominence in recent time; while not a concept addressing the treatment of illness or chronic conditions, its focus is on the prevention of illness.

Consultation with a lifestyle medical practitioner involves open, shared decision-making in an autonomy-supported environment with patients that is respectful of all backgrounds, cultures, and beliefs. Practitioners of lifestyle medicine promote lifestyle as medicine for health promotion, disease prevention, and management of chronic illness and chronic pain conditions. They also address social determinants influencing health. The six pillars of lifestyle medicine are nutrition, sleep, social connections, physical activity, risk reduction, and stress, which are also common themes presented in this book. Now, let us examine how health psychology and adopting a biopsychosocial perspective can help us understand and manage menopause.

HEALTH PSYCHOLOGY – WHAT IS IT?

Health psychology is a topic and a discipline that everyone needs to know about. Why? As life expectancy is increasing, we all would like to live not only longer but in good health, physically and mentally, and enjoy good brain health. Research in the field of health psychology explores our motivations to adopt healthy lifestyle habits to improve and maintain our health. This specialist field of psychology is focused on promoting health as well as the prevention and treatment of disease and illness, in addition to examining how biological, psychological, and social factors influence the choices we make about our health.[6]

One of the primary roles of health psychologists is to empower individuals to make informed decisions about their health. They provide guidance and support in adopting and maintaining health-promoting behaviours. By doing so, they not only improve the physical well-being of individuals but also positively influence their families and contribute to a more productive workforce.

Psychologists are often associated solely with mental health, but in reality, they have a much broader focus. Health psychologists specialise in studying the various factors that contribute to overall well-being, including the ability to maintain good health, recover from illness, and effectively manage chronic conditions. These professionals possess an understanding of the intricate relationship between health and behaviour, which makes them highly sought-after members of interdisciplinary healthcare teams, hospitals, and primary care settings.

Health psychologists also utilise their expertise in other settings, such as private practices, universities, large corporations, government agencies, and specialised clinics. These clinics may focus on areas like oncology, pain management, rehabilitation, smoking cessation, and weight management. By working in these diverse contexts, health psychologists have the opportunity to make a significant impact on the lives of individuals and their families.

A prominent academic and writer in health psychology, Jane Ogden[7] makes the point: given the main causes of death are chronic illnesses such as heart disease, cancer, and diabetes, which are linked to lifestyle choices and behaviours such as eating, drinking alcohol, smoking, and a sedentary lifestyle, behaviour is seen as central to both the onset of illness and its management and therefore is essential to consider this for an individual's health and well-being. Consideration of the psychological and social aspects in menopause does not negate the role of biological factors; it does, however, mean that all three factors are important to provide a more holistic nuanced understanding of menopause symptoms and as a result, provide more tailored targeted individual menopause care to women.

In the biomedical model, diseases are often viewed as resulting from specific biological dysfunction, such as infections, genetic predisposition, or physiological abnormalities. Treatment approaches typically revolve around targeting these underlying biological mechanisms through medication, surgeries or other inventions aimed directly at treating the pathophysiology of the disease. Medical practitioners acknowledge the psychological and social factors as consequences of illness or symptoms, for example, hot flushes and night sweats in menopause may result in low mood, but traditionally, they have failed to consider the role of psychosocial factors as contributing aspects to the onset symptoms and may not fully address the influential aspects of symptoms. Five decades of research within the health psychology field challenge the biomedical model as the influential role of psychosocial factors psychology remains crucial across the health-illness spectrum. This shift recognises behaviour as fundamental to understanding why people fall ill and manage symptoms. It emphasises the importance of addressing health holistically, from prevention to treatment, acknowledging the unique challenges in healthcare. This knowledge is particularly relevant to all stages of menopause.[8]

PSYCHOLOGY AND MENOPAUSE

Although other branches of psychology, such as social psychology, positive psychology, neuropsychology, and clinical and counselling psychology, play a role in promoting health and well-being and can provide valuable insights into the experience and management of menopause. Let us explore how health psychology can help us understand this significant stage in a woman's life.

MEANINGS OF MENOPAUSE

It is crucial to distinguish between the objective 'biological' body and the subjective 'lived experience' that is associated with the distinction between disease and illness. This differentiation allows us to explore the various dimensions of the body and provide a comprehensive understanding of the experience of being ill. Through conducting interviews with women during the peri and postmenopause stages, research in health psychology sheds light on their personal experiences of menopause, providing insights into diverse perspectives and cultural interpretations of this stage of life, as well as its impact on their overall well-being. As mentioned previously, psychology adopts a biopsychosocial approach, which considers other factors in a woman's life, such as life events, psychosocial influences, and cultural contexts.[9]

INDIVIDUAL DIFFERENCES AND PERCEPTIONS

We know from studies in health psychology that our thoughts and perceptions regarding symptoms, as well as the way we assess them and anticipate their effects on us, can significantly influence how we manage and deal with them. When it comes to menopause, psychologists consider a woman's beliefs and attitudes towards this natural process, as well as her cognitive processes, emotional reactions, and behavioural responses to the accompanying symptoms.[10]

ASSESSMENTS AND INTERVENTIONS

Psychologists usually conduct an initial evaluation that helps in identifying mental health difficulties that may arise during menopause. They employ a range of psychological interventions to specifically target symptoms such as depression, anxiety, sleep disturbances, and hot flushes. The research conducted in this field of psychology informs the development of interventions that address the underlying factors contributing to menopause-related symptoms and distress, as well as the overall impact of menopause on well-being and quality of life, with the aim of improving both.[11]

Health psychologists working with a woman going through or a woman who is postmenopausal will take a comprehensive approach, considering the physical and emotional aspects of this stage of life. They recognise that menopause is a complex experience that can have a disruptive impact on women's lives. To effectively manage this inevitable transition, health psychologists focus on various factors such as coping strategies, lifestyle changes, a woman's social support network and psychological well-being.

Psychological support is crucial during this significant life transition. It plays a vital role in helping women navigate the challenges associated with menopause. By providing guidance and assistance, health psychologists empower women to cope with the physical and emotional changes that occur during this phase. Recognising the multifaceted nature of menopause, they offer strategies to manage symptoms and improve overall well-being and quality of life.

The biopsychosocial approach emphasises the interconnectedness of biological, psychological, and social factors in influencing health outcomes. Health psychologists consider the hormonal changes that occur during menopause, the psychological impact of these changes, and the social context in which women experience menopause. This comprehensive perspective allows for a more holistic understanding of menopause and facilitates the development of tailored interventions to support women during this stage of life.

CONCLUSION

In conclusion, the biomedical and biopsychosocial models offer contrasting perspectives on menopause. The biomedical model focuses primarily on the physiological aspects of menopause, whereas the biopsychosocial model considers the interplay of biological, psychological, and social factors. By incorporating health psychology, we gain a deeper understanding of menopause and its management. Health psychology recognises the influence of psychological and social factors on women's experiences of menopause, highlighting the importance of addressing emotional well-being, stress management, and support systems. This perspective emphasises the need for a holistic approach to menopause, considering not only the physical symptoms but also the psychological and social implications.

Furthermore, the biopsychosocial perspective aligns with the concept of lifestyle medicine in managing menopause. Lifestyle medicine recognises that lifestyle choices, such as diet, exercise, and stress management, play a crucial role in overall health and well-being. By adopting a biopsychosocial approach, lifestyle medicine acknowledges that menopause is not solely a physiological event but also an opportunity for women to make positive lifestyle changes that can alleviate symptoms and improve their overall quality of life.

The takeaway message in this chapter is that health psychology and lifestyle medicine provide valuable insights into the understanding and management of menopause. By considering the biopsychosocial perspective, we can address the multifaceted nature of menopause and empower women to take an active role in their health. It is imperative that healthcare professionals, policymakers, and society as a whole embrace this comprehensive approach to menopause, recognising the importance of both physical and psychological well-being throughout this transitional phase in a woman's life and beyond. Decades of research support a biopsychosocial approach to the understanding and management of illness and symptoms, why not adopt this approach to menopause?

NOTES

1   Geraghty (2021).
2   Ogden (2019).
3   Lloyd and Reed (2018).
4   Newson (2019).
5   Hickey et al. (2024).
6   Bolton and Gillett (2019).

7   Ogden (2019).

8   Ogden (2019).

9   Hunter and Smith (2024).

10   Hunter and Smith (2024).

11   Hickey et al. (2024).

3

PSYCHOLOGICAL HEALTH AND BRAIN HEALTH

INTRODUCTION

The journey into menopause usually starts when menstrual cycles become infrequent and irregular and eventually stop altogether, which marks the beginning of the postmenopausal phase. The transition usually takes between two and eight years (with an average of five years) and is characterised by fluctuations in levels of sex hormones. Many women also have vasomotor (constriction or dilatation of blood vessels) symptoms like hot flushes and night sweats, urogenital issues including vaginal dryness and urinary tract infections, as well as a decrease in sexual desire. The transition usually takes place during midlife between the ages of 45 and 55.[1] It's a perfectly natural life stage that often coincides with various other physical health concerns, along with changes in social, professional, and personal roles and other significant life events. That's why menopause is widely seen as a time of significant physical, psychological, and social change.

There has been a growing interest in reported cases of depression among women during the perimenopausal stage of life. This is why it's important for us to identify which women are more likely to develop depression during menopause and to develop targeted preventive measures for them. It's crucial for us to determine whether

DOI: 10.4324/9781003438342-3

the transition into menopause might lead to depression for someone and, if so, what personal and environmental factors might contribute to this risk. It's also important to understand whether the increased risk of depression is limited to the menopause transition itself or if it might persist into the postmenopausal stage.[2]

This chapter will explore the relationship between menopause and depression and discuss the biological, psychological, and social factors that contribute to it. During the perimenopause period, many women not only face psychological distress and stress but also encounter cognitive challenges. These challenges can have a significant impact on their personal and professional lives as they struggle with issues such as difficulty concentrating, memory recall, and an inability to focus on specific tasks. With this in mind, let's look at the importance of maintaining brain health throughout and after menopause and provide practical strategies for mitigating the disruptive phenomenon known as 'brain fog.' Let's also look at the concept of the window of tolerance, which sheds light on how people can regulate their emotional states and at strategies for managing and expanding the window of tolerance to minimise the impact of stress.

In the last ten years, there has been a lot of discussion in both online and print media regarding our mental health and our overall well-being. It's no secret that mental wellness has become a thriving industry, with many people and companies dedicated to promoting it. Maintaining good mental health is crucial, especially during the transition into menopause, as this stage can present unique challenges for women. During this phase of life, it's common to experience low moods, irritability, anxiety, and even depression. However, it's very important to differentiate between occasional feelings of being 'off' or down and clinical depression, which requires a professional diagnosis and treatment.

DEPRESSION

Depression is a widespread condition that can have significant consequences for individuals and their families, friends, and work colleagues. The menopause phase is very often a vulnerable period for the onset of depression, although not every woman will necessarily experience it then. Depression is a global epidemic affecting approximately 350 million people, and its impact is continuously growing. It can deeply affect personal relationships, work productivity, financial stability, and, in extreme cases, even pose a risk of self-harm or suicide. Depression also has severe implications for physical health.[3]

According to the *Diagnostic and Statistical Manual of Mental Disorders* (DSM),[4] depression is defined as an emotional response, a combination of clinical symptoms, and a series of disruptions characterised by a distressing or unpleasant emotional state. This condition is accompanied by difficulties in motor, sensory, and cognitive functioning, a loss of interest or pleasure in previously enjoyable activities (known as anhedonia), a decrease in energy levels, sleep disturbances, reduced libido, and increased feelings of hopelessness.

MENOPAUSE AND DEPRESSION

Throughout history, we've known that menopause can have a major impact on a woman's mental well-being. As far back as the 19th century, medical professionals like French physician Charles Pierre Louis de Gardanne recognised that menopause was linked to psychological distress. This understanding was further advanced in 1959 when Kupperman, Wetchler, and Blatt created the first widely-used checklist for menopause symptoms. This checklist included psychological indicators such as melancholy and nervousness, which showed us the importance of providing mental health support during this time of life.[5]

We all experience times when our mood is less than ideal, and it's a natural part of being human to have fluctuations in our emotional state. Lifetime estimates suggest that around 17% of individuals will experience major depression at some point. However, depression is more prevalent in women – occurring twice as frequently as in men.

It has been widely proposed that women may be at a higher risk of developing depression during times of hormonal changes, such as puberty, pregnancy, and, yes, menopause. Many women commonly report experiencing symptoms of depression and feelings of low mood during this time.[6]

Researchers Vivian-Taylor and Hickey summarised the following research in an article published in 2014. The Pennsylvanian Ovarian Aging Study (PENN Study) involved 436 participants and discovered that during the menopause transition, individuals experienced the highest levels of depressive symptoms compared to both premenopausal and postmenopausal stages. Conversely, the Seattle Midlife Women's Health study, which involved 302 women, found that only the late menopausal transition showed a significant association with an increase in depressive symptoms when compared to pre-menopause. The differences in study design and measures of depressive symptoms like this can impact the results and make it difficult to compare different results from different research. That's why we need to be careful when interpreting the findings and making comparisons. We cannot automatically assume that the presence of depressive symptoms in menopausal individuals indicates an increased risk of depressive disorder. Additionally, the presence of hot flushes, sleep disturbances, sexual dysfunction, and other factors related to depression may further complicate the relationship between depression and menopause.[7]

Three extensive studies in the United States examining the correlation between the transition into menopause and depressive disorder have yielded contradictory findings. The Study of Women's Health Across the Nation (SWAN) is a multicultural longitudinal cohort study investigating women's journey through menopause, and it found that after accounting for psychosocial risk factors and menopausal symptoms, the likelihood of experiencing depressive disorders was twice as high during the menopause transition and nearly four times higher during postmenopause compared to the premenopausal phase. It is worth highlighting that these findings relate to depressive symptoms rather than a formal diagnosis of depressive disorder.

CONTRIBUTING FACTORS TO DEPRESSION IN MENOPAUSE

There can be various reasons for experiencing low mood or depressive symptoms during the transition to menopause and in the early stages of postmenopause. Let's explore some of them:

HORMONAL CHANGES AND MENTAL HEALTH DURING PERIMENOPAUSE

- **Fluctuating hormone levels:** perimenopause brings about significant hormonal changes, including fluctuations in oestrogen and progesterone levels. These changes directly affect the brain and mood, resulting in mood swings, irritability, anxiety and depression. They also have an impact on serotonin levels and on cognitive functioning.[8]
- **Symptoms and risks:** common symptoms of perimenopause, such as irregular periods, hot flushes, night sweats, and sleep disturbances, can exacerbate pre-existing mental health issues.[9]

INFLUENCE OF SOCIETAL AND PERSONAL FACTORS:

- The timing of menopause often coincides with various midlife pressures, such as career demands, caring for elderly parents, and significant life transitions.[10]
- Societal ideals that prioritise youthfulness can have a detrimental effect on self-esteem and body image, further complicating the emotional landscape during perimenopause.
- Various factors, including educational background, rural upbringing, family history of psychiatric illness, and the stage of perimenopause, significantly contribute to anxiety and depression. This

suggests a complex interplay between personal circumstances and mental health.[11]

DEPRESSION RISK FACTORS

Every woman has a different experience of menopause, and the symptoms can vary throughout the stage. It's essential to understand that not all women will encounter mood swings or depression during menopause, but research indicates that certain factors increase the risk of developing mood disorders during it. Women with a history of depression are more likely to experience depressive symptoms during perimenopause; in fact, the incidence of depression doubles, and the risk of developing major depressive episodes increases threefold during this transition compared to the premenopausal stage. During menopause, we need to be aware not only of the potential risk factors associated with mood changes but also of the role of stress in our lives and how we manage it.

STRESS AND DAILY HASSLES

As we discussed earlier, the hormonal changes and health issues that come with menopause can make some women more susceptible to mental health problems. During the perimenopausal stage, about half of all women experience specific anxiety symptoms similar to long-lasting premenstrual symptoms. This stage is also characterised by increased stress, which can be caused by various life events like relationship issues, divorce, the loss of a loved one, or changes in personal, social, family, or work environments. Stress can play a role in triggering or perpetuating disorders such as depression or insomnia. We often hear the phrase "I'm stressed" from friends, family, or colleagues, and we may even use it ourselves from time to time. But what does stress really mean? And how does it differ from the daily irritations and inconveniences we encounter in our lives – our daily hassles? Let's take a look.

While stress and daily hassles are related, they differ in terms of their scope, intensity, and duration. Daily hassles are really the minor annoyances, inconveniences, and challenges that we all encounter in our day-to-day lives. Examples include heavy traffic, road works, household tasks, family issues, or work deadlines. These hassles are relatively short-lived and have a limited impact on our overall well-being.[12]

In contrast, stress encompasses a broader range of experiences and has a more significant impact on our mental and physical health. It involves the body's response to demanding or challenging situations, whether they are acute or chronic. Stress can be triggered by various factors such as work pressure, relationship problems, financial difficulties, or major life changes. Unlike daily hassles, stress tends to be more prolonged and can lead to a variety of symptoms, including irritability, fatigue, difficulty concentrating, and disturbed sleep.[13]

THE DEFINITION OF STRESS

Stress is a combined physiological and psychological response to a perceived threat, challenge, or change. It is a natural reaction that occurs when our bodies and minds interpret a situation as demanding or overwhelming. Stress activates the body's fight or flight mechanism, leading to the release of stress hormones such as cortisol and adrenaline. These hormones prepare our bodies to either confront (fight) the stressor directly or escape from it (flight). The release of these hormones brings on various physiological changes, including an increased heart rate, heightened senses, elevated energy levels, heightened cortisol levels, muscle tension, and alterations in mood and behaviour. If not effectively managed, stress can have both immediate and long-term effects on our health and well-being. Situations are perceived as particularly stressful when they are new, unpredictable, and beyond our control.[14]

CHRONIC STRESS

Chronic emotional stress often brings out feelings of irritability, anger, sadness, a lack of motivation, anxiety, and an overwhelming sense of being burdened. People who are stressed may also exhibit changes in their behaviour, such as an increase in substance abuse or caffeine consumption, social withdrawal, alterations in eating habits (either eating more or less) and/or disruptions in sleep patterns. These behaviours can significantly increase the risk of developing diseases and can even lead to higher mortality rates. Although acute stress can sometimes be beneficial in specific situations, chronic stress or an ongoing negative coping response to stress can have detrimental effects on our overall physical and mental health and quality of life.

Continued exposure to stress hormones over a long period of time can weaken our immune system, making us more vulnerable to illnesses and infections. On top of that, chronic stress can contribute to mental health issues like depression and anxiety. It can also elevate the risk of developing chronic conditions such as cardiovascular disease, diabetes, and certain types of cancer. Some stress arises from the imbalance between the demands of our environment and our personal resources to cope with these demands. The way we see an event as overwhelming or surpassing our capabilities to handle it plays a crucial role in determining the level of stress we experience.

We must recognise the impact that chronic stress can have on our well-being and take proactive steps to manage it effectively. Incorporating stress management techniques into our daily lives, such as practising mindfulness and relaxation exercises, engaging in regular physical activity, seeking support from loved ones or professionals, and adopting healthy coping mechanisms, can significantly improve our overall mental and physical health. By addressing chronic stress head-on and prioritising self-care, we can mitigate its harmful effects and enjoy a healthier and more balanced lifestyle.[15]

STRESS AND MENOPAUSE

Midlife can be an incredibly stressful period for most people, as it often brings about significant life changes. However, studies have shown that there are notable differences between men and women when it comes to experiencing stress. Women tend to report a higher number of stressful life events compared to men, and these events also seem to have a more negative impact on women's well-being.

The SWAN study's comprehensive study of 3,284 participants found that 42% of women reported experiencing moderate levels of stress in the previous week. Additionally, 19% of the study sample reported high levels of stress during the same time frame. It was also discovered that half of the women in the study had undergone one or more stressful life events in the past year.[16]

Similarly, a separate study focused on women in the perimenopausal stage revealed that 40% of participants had encountered at least one very stressful life event in the past six months. These events ranged from divorce or separation to serious illness, the death of a close family member, financial instability, or chronic financial problems[17] It is worth noting that women who experienced menopausal symptoms such as hot flushes also reported feeling more stressed. When women felt more stressed, they also seemed to suffer from more severe menopausal symptoms.

It seems that stress levels tend to be higher among women during midlife, and this can have a profound impact on their overall well-being. The combination of major life changes and the challenges associated with menopause can create a perfect storm of stress for women. Recognising and addressing these stressors is very important in helping support women's health and empowering them to navigate through menopause. By understanding the unique stressors faced by women during midlife, we can work towards creating a society that better supports their mental and emotional well-being.

STRESS MANAGEMENT

Effectively managing and dealing with stress is crucial to dealing with its detrimental effects on our overall health and wellness. There are several strategies that we can use to achieve this, including engaging in regular physical exercise, practising relaxation techniques such as meditation and deep breathing, maintaining a healthy lifestyle through a well-balanced diet, ensuring an adequate amount of sleep, and seeking support from both loved ones and professionals when necessary. It's also very important to address the underlying causes of stress and make any necessary changes in our lives to alleviate its impact.[18]

TREATMENTS AND SOLUTIONS

Despite the advancements in hormone replacement therapies, they are not a one-size-fits-all, universal solution for the challenges that come with menopause. While some women may experience a stabilisation of physical symptoms, it remains crucial to manage and cope with low mood and stress effectively to minimise their negative impact on us.

Fortunately, it's not all bad news about low mood, depression, and stress during menopause. Let's explore a detailed description of the strategies that have been found to be beneficial for women as they approach menopause and navigate life beyond it.

LIFESTYLE MODIFICATIONS

Participate in regular physical activity: Engaging in an exercise regime can assist in diminishing stress hormones and promoting the production of endorphins, which are natural mood enhancers.

Implement relaxation techniques: Deep breathing, meditation, yoga, and progressive muscle relaxation to help calm the mind and alleviate stress.

Maintain a good nutritious diet: Consuming a well-balanced diet abundant in fruits, vegetables, whole grains, and lean proteins can contribute to overall well-being and enhance resilience against stress.

Get enough sleep: Make getting enough quality sleep each night a priority, as sleep deprivation can exacerbate stress levels and negatively impact mood and cognitive function.

COGNITIVE BEHAVIOURAL THERAPY (CBT)

CBT is a widely recognised, evidence-based therapy endorsed by the NICE Guidelines that focusses on the identification and alteration of negative patterns of thinking that contribute to depressive and anxious symptoms and stress. Through CBT, people learn coping mechanisms and strategies to effectively manage stress and depressive and anxious symptoms, including problem-solving techniques, relaxation methods, and cognitive restructuring.[19]

Mindfulness-based stress reduction (MBSR) is a structured programme that incorporates mindfulness meditation, and other mindfulness practises to decrease stress and foster overall well-being. On the course, you can learn to cultivate awareness of the present moment, non-judgemental acceptance and self-compassion, which can aid in reducing reactivity to stressors.

SOCIAL SUPPORT

Engaging with friends, family members, and supportive communities can offer emotional support and practical aid during stressful periods. Sharing one's feelings and experiences with others can help reduce stress and foster a sense of connection. A great move here is to join a menopause support group either online or in person.

PROFESSIONAL COUNSELLING AND PSYCHOTHERAPY

Speaking to a mental health professional like a psychologist, counsellor, or therapist can be really helpful in exploring underlying issues that contribute to stress and developing personalised strategies for coping with depression or anxiety. Therapy sessions may incorporate cognitive behavioural techniques, relaxation training, stress management skills, and an examination of emotional coping mechanisms.

MEDICATION

In some cases, your doctor may prescribe medication to help alleviate the symptoms of stress-related conditions like anxiety and depression. If you experience severe or persistent symptoms, a combination of medications and psychological therapies may be recommended.

Although low mood, depressive symptoms, and stress are common experiences for everyone, it can be particularly challenging for women during and after menopause due to the various demands they face. But don't worry; there are numerous strategies available to manage stress and prevent it from becoming chronic and long-lasting, helping you effectively cope with the daily hassles and stressors that we all inevitably encounter from time to time.[20]

WINDOW OF TOLERANCE

You can get a valuable perspective on stress by considering the 'window of tolerance' model, which is frequently used in the fields of psychology and counselling to explain emotional arousal and responses. The term was originally coined by psychiatrist Daniel Siegel[21] to describe the range of arousal levels at which a person feels comfortable, alert, and capable of functioning effectively. It encompasses a moderate level of arousal that allows individuals to engage with their environment, process information, and adapt to stressors. Within their window of tolerance, people are able to manage stress and regulate their emotions effectively. They exhibit qualities such as flexibility, openness, curiosity, presence, and emotional regulation, which give them the capacity to tolerate life's stressors, maintain a sense of equilibrium, and make adaptive decisions when faced with challenges. On either side of this optimal zone, we find the hyper-arousal zone and the hypo-arousal zone.

According to this concept, when people experience stressors that surpass their capacity to cope, they may move outside their window of tolerance and enter states of hyper-arousal or hypo-arousal.

Hyper-arousal is when they experience overwhelming emotions, such as agitation, anxiety, irritability, or anger. This can be seen through heightened physiological responses like an increased heart rate, muscle tension, and hyper-vigilance. On the other hand, hypo-arousal is when they feel emotionally flat, numb, or disconnected. It is characterised by a decrease in physiological arousal, including a slowed heart rate, reduced sensory awareness, and feelings of emptiness and apathy.

As human beings, we are all unique, and each of us has a distinct and individual perspective influenced by various biopsychosocial factors, personal histories, and experiences. Our backgrounds, temperaments, social supports, and physiology all contribute to our window of tolerance. While it is ideal to stay within our range of optimal emotional states, it is not always realistic. The goal is to expand our window of tolerance and increase our ability to manage our responses to stress and stressors effectively, ultimately cultivating resilience and the ability to quickly return to our optimal zone when we find ourselves outside of it.

Understanding these concepts is essential for anyone seeking to improve their emotional regulation and overall mental health. It empowers us to take control of our emotional experiences and build a healthier relationship with ourselves and others.

How can we maintain or expand our optimal state? A good starting point is to prioritise self-care and actively manage stress in our lives. By developing positive habits and behaviours, as well as identifying and cultivating internal and external resources that promote soothing, regulation, and calmness, we can create a solid foundation. In some cases, seeking guidance from a therapist may be necessary to learn techniques for fostering a healthy, regulated nervous system. Trauma-informed counselling and psychotherapy are specifically designed to help individuals expand their capacity for emotional resilience and self-regulation.[22] Concluding this section on building a healthy nervous system serves as an appropriate segue into the next and final section in this chapter, which explores the topic of brain health.

BRAIN HEALTH

Brain health is a rapidly expanding field, and the World Health Organization has produced a report on optimising brain health throughout life. What is brain health? Basically, it encompasses the ability to maintain and perform mental and physical functions throughout life. It refers to the state of brain functioning across various domains, such as cognitive, sensory, social-emotional, and motor skills, enabling us to reach our full potential over our lifespan. Brain health is about being able to remember, learn, plan, concentrate, and maintain a clear and active mind. It is the state in which our cognitive abilities are at their peak, which can be influenced by our physical health, stress levels, brain function quality, and the lifestyle choices we make. Good brain health means being able to fulfil mental processes and capabilities.[23]

Our brain is an extraordinary organ, weighing approximately one and a half kilos. It regulates everything in our body and keeps our hearts beating and our lungs breathing, but it also defines our identity and gives us the capacity to live, love, learn, laugh, cry, feel, move, and so much more. Taking care of our brains should be a top priority for everyone, especially as we age and for women during and after menopause.

MAINTAINING BRAIN HEALTH

There are various factors that affect brain health, including our physical well-being, the environment in which we live, continuous learning, and social connections, all of which have an impact on the development, adaptability, and response of our brains to stress and difficulties. By recognising and managing these factors, we can optimise our brain health and improve both our mental and physical well-being. However, conditions that affect the brain and nervous system, in general, can arise at any stage of life and are characterised by disruptions in brain growth, damage to brain structure, or impaired brain function.[24]

The human brain, our nervous system's command centre, enables cognition, memory, movement, and emotions through intricate processes – testament to biological evolution. Maintaining optimal brain health is crucial for overall well-being and longevity. As our population ages, the increasing prevalence of neurological disorders poses significant challenges to brain health preservation. Brain health can be influenced by various factors at different stages of life. Have you ever found yourself in a room, unsure why you're there? Perhaps you've struggled to recall names of familiar faces or lost your train of thought mid-sentence. Many women worry these lapses signal early dementia. However, such concerns are common and often unfounded. It's crucial to understand that occasional forgetfulness is normal, especially during times of stress or hormonal changes. Women should prioritise their cognitive health without undue anxiety.

In recent years, there has been a common term circulating called 'brain fog.' For many, it comes as a relief to discover that these symptoms of brain fog can be, but are not limited to, fluctuating or declining hormones.[25]

MENOPAUSE AND BRAIN FOG

The menopausal brain is not just a figment of your imagination. The physical and emotional symptoms that come with hormonal changes are undeniably real and can be incredibly challenging for some women. As we discussed earlier, menopause can often occur simultaneously with other significant life events. It could be your grown children leaving home, the arrival of grandchildren, the onset of chronic illnesses like diabetes or heart disease, the responsibility of caring for ageing parents, planning for retirement, or even a sudden change in your career.

Therefore, any symptoms related to menopause, including its impact on brain function, should be understood within the broader context of your life. In recent years, there has been a lot of talk about brain fog, and many women discuss it on various platforms on social media. This has led to a great deal of speculation as to why some women experience more frequent or severe disruptions in brain functioning than others. Brain fog – possible causes in menopause.

It is possible that oestrogen levels play a role in brain fog. The interaction between hormone levels and neurotransmitters in the brain can also play a part, and this varies from person to person. Also, it has been suggested that engaging in lifelong brain-healthy habits such as intellectual stimulation and physical exercise may offer some protection for cognitive function. During perimenopause and the early stages of menopause, women often report changes in their ability to think clearly, make decisions, and function mentally, where they struggle to absorb and try to make sense of new information.

Research reveals that cognitive decline affects roughly two-thirds of women experiencing menopause or perimenopause. Progesterone decreases first, potentially causing irritability, mood swings, and brain fog. This hormonal shift can disrupt sleep, impacting optimal brain function. The subsequent drop in oestrogen levels leads to classic menopausal symptoms: hot flushes, mood changes, mental confusion, and reduced energy. A University of Rochester[26] study examined 117 middle-aged women, assessing their cognitive function through neuropsychological tests. Researchers evaluated menopausal symptoms and measured hormone levels. Results showed that attention/working memory, verbal learning, verbal memory, and fine motor speed typically decline most significantly in the year following the final menstrual period. This research underscores the profound impact of hormonal changes on women's cognitive health during menopause, highlighting the need for increased awareness and support for women navigating this challenging transition.

While the first year following menopause may be particularly challenging for some women in terms of brain fog, there is hope in the research findings that suggest memory and learning abilities generally return to normal for healthy individuals once the menopause process is complete.

While you wait for menopause to run its course naturally, there are steps you can take to manage the situation. It's important to remember that menopause is also a time for reflection on your health habits and making adjustments that will lead to a healthier middle and old age. In Chapter 7, we'll look at how to develop habits that promote better mental and physical health, as well as brain health. There are ten strategies that you can incorporate into your daily routine to enhance your overall well-being. However, in general, if you're experiencing brain fog, there are several things you can do to help:

1. **Medical check-up**: To start off, it is crucial to undergo a comprehensive health examination and consult your GP to confirm whether your symptoms are indeed linked to menopause or caused by something else. Additionally, it is important to monitor your blood pressure regularly. Elevated blood pressure can trigger hot flushes and also raise the likelihood of experiencing cognitive decline, vascular dementia, and Alzheimer's. Studies have revealed that women with significantly high blood pressure have a 30% higher chance of developing cognitive impairment.

2. **Review your medication**: As you age, there's a higher chance of being prescribed medication for chronic health conditions. Certain types of medication, such as sleeping pills, high blood pressure medications, antidepressants, and statins, may have an impact on your memory and brain function. If you've noticed a decline in your brain function since starting these medications, it's a good idea to ask your doctor or pharmacist to review the medications you're currently taking.

3. **Exercise**: Physical exercise plays a crucial role in preventing chronic illnesses and can also assist in managing irritability, promoting restful sleep, and maintaining a healthy weight and strong bones and muscles. Additionally, both aerobic exercise and resistance training have been shown to impact brain function positively. Just like other bodily structures, the brain relies on good blood flow to function optimally and repair itself. In addition to exercising your body, it is equally important to exercise your mind. Engage in activities that

stimulate your brain, such as making lists to stay organised, challenging yourself with brain teasers or puzzles, reading, studying new subjects, learning a new language, or even playing a musical instrument. Regular social interactions are also beneficial for stimulating the mind. By incorporating both physical and mental exercises into your routine, you can enhance your overall well-being. Not only will you experience the physical benefits of improved health and vitality, but you will also enjoy the cognitive advantages of a sharper mind and increased mental agility.

4. **Sleep**: Sleep can be a constant struggle during the perimenopausal and postmenopausal stages. The quality of sleep is often disrupted, leading to difficulties in cognitive function and contributing to that frustrating brain fog. You should give yourself enough time to wind down and fall asleep while ensuring that your bed and pillows provide maximum comfort and that your bedroom is a serene and dark environment. Avoid having electronic devices in your bedroom that emit light or make noise, as they can prevent you from getting a restful sleep.

5. **Diet**: Taking care of your nutrition involves paying attention to your diet. Make sure you eat a variety of vegetables, fruits, and other unprocessed whole foods, while steering clear of animal fats and trans fats.

6. **Hydration**: When it comes to soft drinks, research has shown that individuals who consume diet drinks are at a higher risk. In fact, those who drink at least one diet drink per day are three times more likely to experience strokes and three times more likely to develop dementia compared to those who don't drink them. Avoid artificial sweeteners like aspartame and choose water to quench your thirst instead.

7. **Alcohol**: A lot of women discover that consuming alcohol during menopause can exacerbate symptoms like hot flushes, night sweats, and insomnia. Alcohol intake has also been linked to increased body weight and elevated blood pressure.

8. **Smoking**: Tobacco has a negative impact on the flow of blood to the brain, which in turn affects brain function. Smoking can also

exacerbate menopausal hot flushes and increase the risk of developing heart and blood vessel disease.

9. **Hormone replacement therapy (HRT)**: Also known as menopause hormone treatment, encompasses a variety of treatments aimed at alleviating menopausal symptoms. HRT can be administered through pills, patches, injections, or implants. However, it is not generally recommended to use HRT as the first-line treatment for menopause-related cognitive issues. We simply don't have enough evidence to show that hormone therapy has positive effects on brain function during menopause, and it is crucial to evaluate both the risks and benefits carefully. The decision to pursue hormone therapy should take into account the severity of cognitive problems and other menopausal symptoms, their impact on your quality of life and work performance, as well as the previous treatment options you have explored.

CONCLUSION

We've seen just how important psychological health and brain health are and recognised the need to prioritise them both throughout and after menopause. We've listed the at-risk subgroups of women for depression, described the concept of brain fog, and offered practical techniques for reducing it.

We also outlined various approaches to maintaining optimal brain health because taking care of your body and mind goes hand-in-hand. It's clear that a depressed mood during the menopausal transition is influenced by various factors and cannot be attributed solely to hormonal changes. Stress, along with its impact on women's lives, plays a significant role. By acknowledging and effectively managing stress, women can enhance their well-being during and after menopause. Understanding the distinction between stress and daily hassles is crucial because it allows us to identify and address the sources of stress in our lives. This includes practising stress-reducing techniques like deep breathing exercises, mindfulness meditation, regular physical activity, and seeking support from loved ones or professionals if necessary. The window of tolerance is crucial for psychological well-being as it represents an optimal zone where individuals can thrive and effectively navigate life's ups and downs. By understanding and expanding our window of tolerance, we can enhance our ability to cope with stress and build resilience. This involves developing self-awareness, learning healthy coping strategies, and seeking support when needed. The window of tolerance gives us a framework for understanding how we can respond to stress and regulate our emotions. By staying within this optimal zone of arousal, we can enhance our capacity to cope with life's challenges and cultivate emotional well-being.

NOTES

1 Newson (2019).
2 Hunter and Smith (2024).
3 Smith (2014).
4 American Psychiatric Association (2013).
5 Muir (2023).
6 Hunter and Smith (2024).
7 Hunter and Smith (2024).
8 Vivian-Taylor and Hickey (2014).
9 Vivian-Taylor and Hickey (2014).
10 Vivian-Taylor and Hickey (2014).
11 Vivian-Taylor and Hickey (2014).
12 Rohleder (2019).
13 Wright et al. (2018).
14 Wright et al. (2018).
15 Antonovsky (2002).
16 Hickey et al. (2024).
17 Hickey et al. (2024).
18 Antonovsky (2002).
19 Percival (2023).
20 Percival (2023).
21 Siegel (2010).

22 Stanley (2019).
23 Mosconi (2024).
24 Mosconi (2024).
25 Mosconi (2024).
26 Weber et al. (2013).

4

THE SELF IN TRANSITION

INTRODUCTION

Menopause signifies a significant transition in a woman's life, indicating the end of her reproductive years and the beginning of a new stage in older adulthood. This pivotal phase profoundly impacts a woman's perception of herself, her identity, self-worth, and body image.[1] As women navigate through the physical and psychological changes associated with menopause, they are confronted with a complex interplay of personal narratives and societal influences that shape how they view themselves. This chapter explores how our personal identity is moulded by the experiences we encounter throughout our lives, as well as the role played by social identity in shaping our sense of self. We will explore how our identity is influenced by both our genetic makeup and the social environment we inhabit, including the people we interact with in our social network. Additionally, we will provide explanations for key concepts such as self-esteem, self-concept, body image, and the ageing self. The aim of this chapter is to emphasise the fluid nature of self-concept, identity, and body image, particularly in relation to women in midlife and beyond. We are, in essence, a self in transition.

DOI: 10.4324/9781003438342-4

THE SELF AND PERSONHOOD

One of the pioneers in the field of modern psychology, William James (1842–1910), characterised the self as a dynamic process of understanding and cognition involving two aspects: the subject (referred to as "I," representing self-reflective acts) and the object (known as "me," representing the self-awareness of oneself).[2] According to James, there are three dimensions of the self: the material self (which includes our physical body and possessions), the social self (which involves our perception of how others see us), and the spiritual self (which encompasses our personality and psychological aspirations).[3] The concept of "the self" has been extensively explored in literature, focusing on questions such as how we shape our identity and how menopause impacts our sense of self. It is crucial to engage in discussions about our notions of self, including self-identity, self-concept, self-esteem, and body image, as these topics often arise in conversations about menopause. However, it is essential to question whether we truly grasp the meaning behind these terms. We may have vague ideas about these concepts, so let's explore these concepts from the field of social psychology.

SELF-IDENTITY

A fundamental aspect of being conscious is having a sense of self or identity. We are aware of being unique individuals with our own distinct personas. This arises from our interaction with the world as well as our deep understanding of our inner thoughts and emotions. Our sense of self, often referred to as "I," is derived from our awareness of who we are.

One way to conceptualise a person's identity is by considering it as a combination of personal identity and social identity. Personal identity is formed through our individual experiences and personal reflections on them. On the other hand, social identity refers to the characteristics and roles that others assign to us. It encompasses how society perceives and defines us.[4]

Our personal identity is shaped by the unique experiences we have throughout our lives. These experiences, along with our own introspection, contribute to the development of our sense of self. They form the foundation upon which our personal identity is built.

In addition to personal identity, social identity plays a significant role in shaping who we are. It encompasses the aspects of ourselves that are defined by our interactions with others and the social groups we belong to. Society often assigns us certain roles and attributes based on factors such as our gender, ethnicity, occupation, or social status. These external labels can influence how we perceive ourselves and how others perceive us.

Ultimately, our sense of self is a complex interplay between our personal experiences and the way society perceives us. It is a dynamic process that evolves over time as we navigate through life and interact with others. Understanding and embracing both our personal and social identities allows us to have a more comprehensive understanding of ourselves and the world around us.

One of the key aspects of being self-aware is our ability to engage in introspection, step back, and reflect on our experiences. We can actively choose to be aware and mindful of our thoughts, actions, and choices; we are autonomous human beings with personal agency. This self-awareness becomes especially valuable for women in midlife, as it presents an opportune moment to reflect on various aspects of life, such as personal decisions, relationships, health, and lifestyle. Our capacity for self-reflection also involves the power to imagine alternative paths and possibilities, recognising that change is possible while acknowledging that certain aspects of our lives and ourselves may remain unchanged.

In this way, we don't view life as fixed and unchangeable. Instead, we embrace the potential for transformation in how we perceive ourselves and respond to challenges like menopause symptoms, illness, and the ageing process. We possess the ability to learn new strategies for addressing both old and new problems. This is particularly relevant for women approaching menopause or those in the postmenopausal stage of life.

SELF-CONCEPT

As we explore the depths of our individuality and our self-concept, it is crucial to acknowledge the impact of our social surroundings. After all, no one exists in isolation. Our perception of ourselves, commonly referred to as our self-concept, is shaped by a myriad of factors. For instance, a child might define themselves by their age, proudly proclaiming "I am six years old." Similarly, a woman in the middle stages of life might describe herself in relation to one of several roles of parent, grandparent, partner, employed, or unemployed or refer to herself as menopausal. It is important to note that we are not born with a self-concept; rather, it evolves throughout our lifespan and varies from person to person. It is influenced by both internal and external forces.[5]

Our self-concept encompasses various aspects of our identity. Some facets are consciously chosen, such as our chosen career path, while others are innate and bestowed upon us, like our nationality. The combination of these different components shapes our understanding of who we are.[6]

Self-concept is the way in which we understand ourselves. It encompasses our physical and moral perceptions, as well as how we assess ourselves. Our self-identity plays a significant role in shaping our self-concept. The components of our self-concept, known as self-schemas, are the specific beliefs that define who we are. These schemas serve as mental frameworks through which we organise our understanding of ourselves and the world around us. When it comes to menopause, our self-concept can either portray us as experienced women filled with wisdom, vibrancy, and enthusiasm for the future or as individuals who believe they are past their prime, lacking expectations for the future. Our self-concept greatly influences how we process, remember, and evaluate both ourselves and others. Ultimately, the notion of self-concept seeks to answer the fundamental question, "Who am I?"[7]

SELF-ESTEEM

Our perception of ourselves is influenced by two key factors: self-esteem and social comparisons. Self-esteem refers to how we evaluate ourselves, both positively and negatively. When we have high self-esteem, we hold ourselves in high regard, recognising our value, abilities, and worth. On the other hand, low self-esteem involves harsh judgements based on past experiences and low expectations for future accomplishments. If someone sees themselves as intelligent, competent, and well-adjusted, they likely have high self-esteem. Conversely, if they believe they are unintelligent, incompetent, and poorly adjusted, their self-esteem is low. It's important to note that self-esteem can fluctuate depending on social situations and different stages of our lives.[8]

Another aspect of our self-concept is self-worth. This is derived from our confidence in what we do and our beliefs and behaviours. As early as 1902, Cooley introduced the concept of the "looking glass self." This theory suggests that we base our sense of self on how we think others perceive us. By using social interactions as a mirror, we rely on the judgements and feedback we receive from others to gauge our worth, values, and behaviour.

Additionally, theorists in social psychology introduce us to the concept of social comparisons. This idea highlights how we tend to compare ourselves to others to evaluate our own abilities and attributes. By observing others' achievements or characteristics, we gain insight into our own strengths and limitations.

BEING A PERSON

Now that we have covered the formal definitions of the concept of 'self,' let's explore what it truly means to be a person. As human beings, we are more than just a collection of physiological enzymes and functions or instinctual behaviours. Each of us exists within a unique social sphere shaped by our lived experiences. We are not only aware of our own existence, but we are also perceived by others as individuals with distinct backgrounds, behaviours, and expectations for the future.

Being a person encompasses the idea of embodiment, being connected to a specific physical form. It involves subjective experiences, consciousness, a sense of self, personal identity, self-perception, and the capacity to initiate thoughts and actions. It also encompasses our thoughts, perceptions, and the way we make sense of information and experiences. To be a person is to exist in relation to others within a social context defined by shared meanings and customs. It involves unconscious emotions and the recognition that some of our reactions and experiences stem from deep-rooted feelings within ourselves, even if we are not fully conscious of them. Being a person entails acknowledging the uniqueness and individuality of yourself and others.[9]

Being a person means embracing our humanity in all its complexity and nuance. It means recognising that we are more than just biological beings; we are social creatures who thrive on connection and understanding. Being a person means navigating the intricate web of relationships, emotions, and experiences that shape our lives. It means being open to growth, change, and self-discovery. Ultimately, being a person is about embracing our individuality while recognising the common threads that bind us all together as human beings.

EMBODIMENT

As a human being, embodiment is of utmost importance. Our body serves as the vessel for our experiences, skills, communication, and relationships. It is through our bodies that we exist as individuals, and it comes as no surprise that the way it functions or malfunctions can greatly impact our overall experience. We witness this phenomenon regularly – menopausal symptoms, illness, or medication can all have significant effects on our emotional well-being, our ability to connect with others, and even our sense of self. These changes, in turn, influence the quality of our lives. This becomes particularly evident as we approach menopause and navigate the various changes in our bodies, psychological states, emotional responses, and shifting perspectives on our identity within a changing social context. The physical body not only allows us to experience sensations and sensual pleasure but also exposes us to disease and pain. This is especially true during ageing, where physical issues remind us of the transient nature of life itself.[10]

Our existence as human beings is deeply intertwined with our social interactions. How people perceive and respond to us can greatly influence our self-concept. This becomes especially relevant during menopause when physical changes such as weight gain, dry skin, and dry hair can impact our body image. Research has shown that our sense of physical attractiveness, or our belief that we are no longer attractive or desirable, is not solely determined by our own physical traits but also by how others interact with us and the opinions they hold of us. The way others react to and perceive our physical characteristics plays a significant role in shaping our own beliefs about ourselves.

BODY IMAGE

Puberty and pregnancy are typically seen as times of positive change and growth. However, menopause is often associated with negative stereotypes, portraying women as depressed, sick, and unattractive. Menopause signifies the shift from a woman's reproductive years to her non-reproductive years and can be viewed as the transition from youth to older adulthood. Like other hormone-related life transitions, this physical change can influence a woman's self-concept and body image and potentially affect her health behaviours, social interactions, and overall quality of life.[11]

The philosophy of Merleau-Ponty, in his work from 1962, centres on the idea that human beings are embodied entities.[12] This suggests that our body serves as a medium through which we perceive the world around us. It is when our body malfunctions or experiences symptoms that we become particularly aware of it as a physical entity. This heightened awareness of the physical self can be attributed to both cultural influences and individual differences in our bodies compared to others.

Body image encompasses the psychological experience of being embodied, involving perceptions of the body's appearance and abilities. It is influenced by various factors, such as societal standards, personal beliefs, and individual experiences. Considering a woman's body image, health, and chronic conditions throughout her lifespan is crucial to providing appropriate support and interventions during menopause. Taking a biopsychosocial approach allows for a comprehensive understanding of the biological, individual, and social aspects involved in menopausal support.

Understanding the significance of the body as an integral part of our perceptions and experiences allows for a more comprehensive approach to supporting women during menopause. In this way, menopause, according to research, can be closely linked to the ageing process. This connection often leads to a conflict between how one perceives themselves externally, as someone who is growing older and potentially less vibrant, and how they feel internally, where they still see themselves as youthful and eager to embrace the next stage of, consequently, menopause can significantly impact a person's self-concept and self-esteem.

How an individual experiences the transition through menopause largely depends on their own evaluation of this complex biographical disruption and the coping mechanisms they employ to navigate it. The emotional toll of a changing body image can intensify the effects of menopause, with women who experience more vasomotor symptoms often reporting heightened catastrophising thoughts and negative self-perceptions. However, feeling in control of these symptoms can help alleviate their impact.

Health care providers offering a range of medical and psychological menopause treatment options will help empower women to take control of their own health by choosing which interventions to adopt and when. In a similar vein, as discussed by O'Donnell and Habenicht (2021)[13] regarding illness self-concept, these interventions may also help women adjust to a new sense of self and identity. By embracing these practises, women can explore their autonomy and personal agency in managing their menopausal experience.

Our ability to reflect on our lives and remember gives us a sense of continuity in our experiences. As a result, our conscious awareness is shaped by our thoughts, ways of thinking, and emotions. This enables us to assign meaning to events and take responsibility for our actions, whether they are positive or negative. It helps us navigate the world and maintain a sense of control. The style and complexity of this cognitive framing vary from person to person. Throughout our daily lives, our conscious awareness undergoes constant changes. Factors such as education, intelligence, and values, which are influenced by the social context we live in, contribute to these changes.

A fundamental aspect of being human is our belief in our ability to take action and make things happen. This is known as personal agency. When it comes to menopausal symptoms, we have the power to seek guidance, support, and help whenever we feel the need. We have the autonomy to become informed and make decisions that are in our best interest. Autonomous agency refers to the extent to which individuals are capable of independent actions, doing things because they believe it is the right course of action for themselves.

SELF IN TRANSITION

By utilising the concept of linguistic repertoire, we can connect it to the entirety of our life stories. The true meaning of menopause is therefore understood through our own introspection, or, in other words, the self as an observer. When we try to make sense of something, we reconstruct our self-concept and personal histories based on recent and current events. Additionally, when we seek to understand the experiences of others, we rely on the narratives they share with us.

Our individuality and unique self-identity are shaped in part by the narratives we construct to make sense of ourselves and our origins. These narratives are influenced by our culture and the meanings we attribute to them, but they also play a role in reshaping and redefining those meanings. We become acutely aware of this process when we introduce ourselves to others for the first time. It is during these moments that we recognise the fluidity of our self-concept.

This becomes particularly evident as we undergo changes in our self-concept, identity, and self-esteem during midlife. It is important to acknowledge that women in midlife and beyond are constantly evolving and transforming themselves. We are, in essence, a self in transition.

SELF AND OTHERS

Let's reflect on the impact of other individuals and the social environment on shaping and maintaining our identity. People play a significant role in our personal lives, even when they are not physically present. We keep them close through photographs, phone calls, videos, and social media connections. Our lives are intertwined with others most of the time.

Just as our bodies provide the vessel for our existence, the social world also shapes the type of person we are or aspire to be. Our social practises and modes of communication, acquired from our surroundings, form the foundation of our identity. These influences shape how we perceive ourselves and how we present ourselves to others.[14]

Our sense of self is shaped by the way others perceive and respond to us. Their categorisation of us determines how we see ourselves. Understanding the expectations associated with our identity helps us navigate how we should behave, react, and even how we should think and feel.

It's important to recognise that, as human beings, our experiences are not solely based on thoughts or cognitions. In Chapter 3, we discovered that as women approach menopause, they often experience low mood, mood swings, and irritability. This can also continue into the postmenopause stage of life. Our feelings and emotions, such as excitement, hostility, happiness, or boredom, play a significant role and can sometimes be pervasive, protracted, and overwhelming. These emotions have the power to shape our daily experiences and have an impact on our self-concept and self-esteem. However, understanding the origins of these feelings and being consciously aware of them can be a challenge. Sometimes, our feelings may seem to arise from deep within us, beyond the boundaries of our conscious understanding.

TIME

The concept of time holds significant importance at this juncture. We have discovered that our biological makeup intertwines with social factors, thus impacting our sense of self. Our memories, both conscious and unconscious, have the power to shape how we perceive ourselves in the present moment and influence our hopes and fears for the future. Each individual possesses a unique sense of personal biological continuity. While there is a continuous thread that connects us throughout the decades, change is also inevitable. Age serves as a prominent and often unspoken marker of our identity. Growing older is not just a biological process; it is equally a social phenomenon. Our expectations and attitudes towards ourselves and others may be influenced by societal assumptions about ageing and, more specifically, menopause.

Furthermore, there exists a deep existential mystery that underpins our existence as individuals. While we may possess a certain degree of autonomy to make choices and determine our actions, it is important to acknowledge that the person we ultimately become is shaped by factors beyond our control. We do not have the power to choose our parents, the body we inhabit, or the society in which we were raised. In fact, we had no say in being born in the first place.

THE AGEING SELF

As this chapter draws to a close, a key takeaway message is that the self holds the key to finding meaning in life, especially as we age. The awareness of our mortality becomes a major concern as we grow older. Numerous studies have shown that the physical and psychological changes that accompany menopause can challenge a woman's sense of identity, self-esteem, and body image. However, it is not all doom and gloom. Throughout adulthood, setting personal goals can bring about a renewed sense of vitality while reducing feelings of apathy. Vitality is closely tied to qualities such as self-reliance, energy, resilience, and an overall improvement in quality of life. On the other hand, apathy is linked to low self-esteem, dependence, boredom, lethargy, and a diminished quality of life.[15]

While ageing and menopause are inevitable, setting age-appropriate goals can significantly enhance our quality of life and lead to better psychological well-being compared to not setting goals or setting minimal or inappropriate ones. The concept of ageing is evolving, as highlighted in Chapter 6 where we explore the research which shows us that people are living longer and remaining active well into later life. This shift in perspective allows us to reconstruct the model of ageing in later life, empowering the ageing self to embrace new possibilities and experiences and to build and enhance self-esteem and self-concept regardless of age or menopausal status.

CONCLUSION

In conclusion, this chapter explored the intricate journey of self, shedding light on the multifaceted nature of personal identity. It emphasises that our self-concept and self-esteem are not static but rather fluid, influenced by our perception of how others perceive us. Menopause acts as a catalyst for self-reflection and introspection as women cope with physical and emotional changes. The chapter explored the significance of understanding ourselves in this transitional phase, highlighting the importance of embracing our evolving selves and challenging societal norms. By recognising that our self-concept is shaped by both internal and external factors, we can cultivate a stronger sense of self and enhance our self-esteem. This chapter serves as a reminder that menopause is not solely a biological process but also a transformative experience that offers an opportunity for self-discovery and growth. It calls for a compassionate and supportive social network that empowers women to redefine their identities beyond traditional roles and expectations. By embracing the fluidity of self during and after menopause, we can foster a culture that champions women's autonomy, agency, and well-being. This chapter serves as an empowering resource, urging women to embrace their unique journey to understand the complexities of self at midlife and beyond.

NOTES

1 Muir (2023).
2 Pennington (1986).
3 Myers (2023).
4 Myers and Spencer (2006).
5 Myers and Spencer (2006).
6 Pennington (1986).
7 Stevens (1996).
8 Pennington (1986).
9 Stevens (1996).
10 Stevens (1996).
11 Stevens (1996).
12 Froman (2000).
13 O'Donnell and Habenicht (2021).
14 Myers (2023).
15 Arnould et al. (2013).

5

SEXUAL WELL-BEING DURING AND AFTER MENOPAUSE

INTRODUCTION

Sexual well-being, both during and after menopause, is a very important part of women's health and overall quality of life. In this chapter, I'd like to move beyond the traditional focus on sexual dysfunction and hormonal changes and instead explore the many factors that influence our sexuality in midlife. With women spending a significant part of their lives in the postmenopausal period, addressing sexual well-being is crucial. Also, as life expectancy continues to rise and new and different treatments become available, prioritising sexual well-being in menopause care becomes a critical part of our lives. In this chapter, we will explore some of the factors that impact sexual functioning and overall well-being for women in midlife. I hope I can help you understand sexual well-being within a biopsychosocial framework, encompassing not only physical health but also pleasure and psychosocial elements such as the dynamics of relationships and sexual self-esteem. By promoting a sex-positive mindset and reshaping the narrative around sexual experiences at midlife, women can reclaim independence and control of their sexual well-being during and after menopause. In discussing sexual health at this life stage, I hope you'll gain a broader perspective

DOI: 10.4324/9781003438342-5

that encompasses not just dysfunction but also overall sexual health and well-being. We must acknowledge that sexual pleasure and satisfaction are influenced by a number of factors, including the physical, emotional, and social dimensions of sexual experiences and the ability to find intimacy with a partner. Let's explore just how common sexual issues are for women through menopause and examine the various factors contributing to sexual difficulties. We can take a look at potential solutions for enhancing sexual functioning and well-being among women in midlife and beyond. By helping to recognise the impact of social conditions and life stressors on sexual desire, I want to provide some valuable insights and guidance for healthcare professionals and women navigating this transformative stage of life. As we address aspects of sexual well-being, we can broaden the conversation around menopausal sexual health and offer comprehensive support for women and healthcare providers alike.

SEXUAL HEALTH AND SEXUAL WELL-BEING

Sexual health is a key indicator of overall well-being and life satisfaction. For women, engaging in fulfilling sexual activities significantly impacts their physical, mental, and relational wellness. However, many women face substantial obstacles to their sexual function throughout their lives, necessitating attention and support. A study found that between 42% and 68% of middle-aged women are sexually active, and of those, 42% to 88% experience sexual dysfunction at some point.[1]

Sexual health is affected by a number of things, including personal factors, interpersonal relationships, social and family dynamics, and culture. According to the *Diagnostic and Statistical Manual of Mental Disorder* (9DSM-5), sexual dysfunction is defined as "a disturbance in the sexual response cycle or pain associated with sexual intercourse."[2] The prevalence of sexual dysfunction among women is estimated at between 25% and 63%. In postmenopausal women, that number is higher, with rates between 68% and 86%.[3]

Sexual issues that cause distress and last for six months or more are classified as dysfunction by the DSM. Studies on middle-aged and older women show mixed results about how age, menopause, and partner status affect sexual activity and function. While some research suggests that sexual problems increase with age, other studies link ageing to overall health declines that impact sex, including chronic illnesses like diabetes and heart conditions and medications like beta-blockers that negatively impact sexual function. As women age, their sexual health deserves attention and care. We must challenge assumptions about sexuality in later life and advocate for comprehensive healthcare that addresses women's unique needs. By understanding these complex factors, we can better support women's sexual well-being throughout their lives.

SEXUAL FUNCTION ACROSS THE LIFESPAN

Research tells us that sexual activity and well-being remain crucial for women's overall well-being, regardless of age. Contrary to misconceptions, ageing doesn't eliminate sexual desires; it may simply alter how they are expressed. Many older women seek both sexual and emotional intimacy, while some prefer one or the other. It's important to recognise that some women may choose to forgo these connections entirely. Understanding and respecting these diverse needs are essential for promoting holistic health and empowerment among older women.

It is important to dispel the myth that older adults are not interested in sex. Research tells us the truth here: Janine Steckenrider summarises the research in this area; in a UK study, 86% of men and 60% of women aged 60 to 69 years said they were sexually active, as did 59% of men and 34% of women aged 70 to 79 years, and 31% of men and 14% of women aged 80 years and older. That is a pretty good cause for optimism. Another study from Sweden found that 10% of people older than 90 years reported being sexually active.

In a study in the United States, of people who were sexually active, aged 75 to 85 years, 54% reported having sex two to three times per week, and 23% reported having sex one or more times per week. In the Retired Persons' Healthy Ageing Poll of individuals aged 65 to 80 years, two-thirds said they were interested in sex, and more than 50% said sex was important to their quality of life.[4]

Sex is a core aspect of human life, including sexuality, gender identity, sexual orientation, libido, pleasure, and intimacy. We've looked at the statistics from the UK, and other studies support those figures – 42% of women and 60% of men aged 65–74 years have an active sexual life.[5]

The postmenopausal period is marked by physical and psychological changes for women. When there are major symptoms, this phase can have a negative impact on sexuality, which has led to menopause being associated with sexual dysfunction for many people.[6]

Studies confirm that maintaining an active sexual life is crucial, particularly as we age. Physically, regular sexual activity enhances circulation, skin elasticity, and joint flexibility. It also promotes general health. Engaging in sex on a regular basis contributes to overall physical well-being. Having a fulfilling sexual life is not just pleasurable but also beneficial for our long-term health and vitality.

From a psychological perspective, sex is largely the inevitable result of the development of love, connection, and intimacy. It increases our vitality and enriches the content and quality of our lives, so it is also true that sex keeps you psychologically healthy.

Research indicates that sexual activity significantly impacts the overall well-being of older adults. Post-orgasm prolactin release in the brain helps reduce stress and anxiety, contributing to an improved mental health. Satisfying sexual experiences are proven to be effective in managing these issues. Studies confirm that the desire for sexual and emotional intimacy in relationships persists with age. For older adults, a fulfilling sex life provides crucial emotional and social support within relationships and helps provide a basis for positive ageing.[7]

SEXUAL FUNCTIONING IN WOMEN IN MENOPAUSE

In general, however, sexual activity declines as we get older, and for women, there has been a lot of debate on the impact of menopause on this part of their lives. Sexual function and its influencing factors remain highly debated. Research on the impact of menopause on sexuality yields conflicting results. Some studies suggest a negative effect, while others indicate the opposite. Many women view menopause as a liberating phase for their sex lives, free from pregnancy concerns and bolstered by long-term relationships. However, individual experiences vary greatly. Research has identified several sexual issues that some menopausal women face, including reduced sexual desire, less frequent sexual activity, decreased sexual response, orgasm difficulties, and diminished genital sensitivity. Other studies have found that interpersonal factors affect sexual function.[8] It is crucial to recognise that each woman's journey through menopause is unique, and their sexual experiences during this time can differ significantly.

A word of caution about these research findings. It is difficult to find definitive answers in relation to this as women attending menopause specialist clinics often report problems related to sexual functioning. We cannot make generalised statements about sexual functioning from this research, and we also know that fewer than half of menopausal women seek menopause-related treatment, and those who do, tend to report more life stress and clinical depression, anxiety and psychological symptoms, all of which relate to sexual functioning.

Research from the general population is mixed, as some studies with menopausal women do not show clear associations between menopause and reduced levels of sexual functioning. Other studies have found women in midlife to have lower sexual interest among peri-menopausal and postmenopausal women compared with pre-menopausal women.

Menopause brings hormonal shifts that impact sexual health. Lower oestrogen and androgen levels can alter sexual organs and bodily systems, affecting sexual function. Studies confirm that declining oestrogen levels are linked to reduced sexual function. Androgen levels, particularly testosterone, have also been studied. Lower testosterone levels are seen as predictors of sexual dysfunction, especially in women experiencing natural menopause. These findings highlight the complex interplay between hormones and sexual health during and after menopause, emphasising the need for comprehensive women's health care.

It has also been shown that the use of HRT has a positive effect on the sexual function of menopausal women, with strong evidence showing it significantly improves sexual function. But it is also important to consider other factors, some we can change and some we cannot, that contribute to sexual function and sexual well-being.

CONTRIBUTING FACTORS TO SEXUAL DIFFICULTIES IN MENOPAUSE

Several studies have addressed the many factors (including physical, psychological and social factors) impacting sexual function in menopausal women. Let's take a look at the research findings in these areas:[9]

Physical issues include:

- The age of the woman and her partner
- Hormonal changes
- Duration of perimenopause
- Type of menopause (surgical or natural)
- Chronic illness, partner's illness or poor health
- Partners sexual problems
- Severity of physical menopausal symptoms, including vasomotor symptoms (hot flushes, night sweats)
- Physical activity
- Medications
- Obstetric history
- General health status

Psychological and emotional factors include:

- Depression
- Anxiety
- Attitude towards sexuality
- Attitude and feelings toward sexual partner
- Quality of the relationship
- Duration of the interpersonal relationship
- Level of self-confidence, self-esteem, and body image

So, sexual function and sexual well-being are influenced by a variety of factors, some of which we can modify and others we can't. One particular issue that frequently arises in research and therapy is the sexual self-esteem of women during and after middle age. This issue is so prevalent that it deserves to be addressed here.

SEXUAL SELF-ESTEEM

Sexual self-esteem can be influenced and moulded by various life experiences. For some women, the changes that occur in their bodies during menopause can lead to negative emotions and a sense of self-consciousness during sex. This may result in avoiding sexual encounters, difficulties in experiencing arousal and achieving orgasm, and even hesitancy in discussing how you feel or when sexual activity becomes painful or uncomfortable.

Sexual self-esteem encompasses five key components.[10] Take a moment to reflect on your own sexual encounters and if there is potential for growth and increased confidence in these areas for you.

- **Skill and expertise**: The ability to desire and be desired by a sexual partner, as well as being open to sexual opportunities.
- **Appeal**: The perception of your own sexual attractiveness, regardless of how others see you, and having confidence in your own beauty and appeal.
- **Control**: The capability to guide and manage your thoughts, emotions, and sexual interactions.

- **Moral judgement**: Alignment between your thoughts, feelings, and sexual behaviours with your own moral principles. Moral judgement also involves the capacity to self-assess thoughts, emotions, and sexual conduct.
- **Adaptability**: Harmony or compatibility between your experiences and sexual behaviours with your personal objectives or aspirations. This entails being able to adjust your sexual behaviour to align with the goals of others.

Several situations can negatively impact your sexual self-esteem, such as past unpleasant sexual encounters, illness, cancer, and subsequent treatment, as well as physical disabilities. If you're struggling with your sexual self-esteem, it is important to talk to your partner, GP, or a professional therapist for support.

You might be familiar with a pattern of thinking or behaviour called 'spectatoring,' which refers to the tendency of women with a negative body image to focus on the perceived flaws of their bodies during sexual experiences. Many women who struggle with their sexual self-esteem experience this.

Spectatoring can be a distraction that leads us to avoid sexual activity and decreases sexual satisfaction, which can affect arousal and orgasm. It becomes challenging to fully engage in the present moment and enjoy fulfilling sexual experiences when you are preoccupied with your perceived physical imperfections and viewing your body from an external perspective. In other words, you can't fully enjoy sex when you're worried about how the other person sees your body.[11]

For women going through menopause, dealing with chronic health issues or pain, or having physical disabilities, sexual self-esteem can become even more complex. Additionally, women who have survived cancer may face challenges in accepting and adapting to their post-treatment bodies. It's really, really important to acknowledge these complexities and get support from healthcare professionals or therapists who specialise in these issues.

Remember that addressing and improving your sexual self-esteem is a journey that requires patience and self-compassion.

By getting help and practicing self-care, you can work towards developing a healthier and more positive relationship with your body and sexuality.

Although there are various elements that can have a negative impact on your body confidence and sexual self-esteem, there are ways to improve both aspects. Factors that can positively influence your sexual self-esteem encompass the recognition and acceptance of your evolving body image, both on your own and by your partner, fostering strong emotional connections, and cultivating a positive perception of your own attractiveness.

To enhance your self-esteem and sexual self-esteem, think about the following suggestions offered by Rydberg and Vegunata from the Mayo Clinic Women's Health Department:[12]

Make it a priority to nurture yourself with gentleness and empathy, fully embracing and accepting your true self. Inform yourself of sexual well-being and learn more about how to promote a positive body perception. Be aware of any negative habits that might impede your sexual experience, such as spectatoring.

When it comes to your inner voice, it's important to remember that you should treat yourself as you would treat a close friend. Instead of feeling ashamed or apologetic about our sexual needs and desires, we should fully embrace body and sex positivity. Learn ways to be confident and assertive, discard self-doubt, and find your voice in expressing what feels right and pleasurable to you.

Surround yourself with people who bring positivity and encouragement into your life. It is important to appreciate and accept compliments. It is essential to establish boundaries and confidently say 'no' when you need to. By surrounding yourself with uplifting and supportive individuals, you can cultivate a healthy sense of self-worth and foster a positive impact on your overall well-being.

Recognising, understanding, and expressing your emotions is also important, as it allows for open and honest communication with others. If you are in a relationship, it is important to engage in conversations that are open and honest about your and your partner's sexual needs and desires. While it may be a little uncomfortable, it is important to have conversations about taboo areas of sexuality while respecting each other's boundaries.

Discover the power of establishing daily rituals and behaviours that foster a mindset conducive to intimacy (learn more about habit formation in Chapter 7). Become informed with accurate and reliable trusted information about sexuality. Engage in reading educational resources, such as informative books on this topic, to expand your understanding of yourself and your connections with others. By deepening your awareness, you can enrich your relationships and ignite a sense of passion. Embrace the opportunity to cultivate habits that not only nurture your personal growth but also empower you to embrace your sexuality confidently. It would be useful to consider sensate focus exercises, either alone or with a partner – for more details on sensate focus, see page 125 in Further Reading and Websites chapter.

SEX POSITIVITY

The World Health Organization recognises that sexual pleasure and intimate relationships are essential human rights. As a society, we should no longer consider sex as a deviant behaviour that requires justification but rather as a positive and affirming expression of celebration. Recent research studies consistently show that maintaining a positive attitude towards sexuality is closely linked to experiencing higher levels of sexual satisfaction. This, in turn, has a profound impact on various aspects of our well-being, including social, emotional, physical, and mental health.

In addition to these significant benefits, embracing a sex-positive mindset gives us lots of other advantages. For example, people who adopt this approach report reduced sexual anxiety, including concerns related to performance. Furthermore, they experience improved sexual functioning, with a particular emphasis on the pursuit of pleasure, whether it is enjoyed alone or with a partner. Consequently, this can lead to enhanced sexual esteem and an overall boost in self-confidence.

Unsurprisingly, *The Psychology of Menopause* emphasises the central role of our beliefs and attitudes, which play a crucial role in shaping our behaviour and emotional responses to menopause experience. So, it's fitting to say that sex starts in the mind as our beliefs and attitudes shape our sexual behaviour and experiences. It's essential and timely at this point to explore the concept of sex positivity, which involves adopting a liberating attitude towards sexuality, free from shame and judgement.

In the past, societal norms heavily influenced by religious beliefs often treated sex and sexuality as taboo subjects, as indeed menopause once was too. Fortunately, this mindset has changed over the years. This belief system created a culture of stigma that perpetuated harmful and regressive views on something that is a natural and integral part of being human. We have also learned in chapter one that historically, women were cast aside when past their reproductive stage of life and, therefore, by default, were not considered useful, desirable, or attractive. Contemporary societies struggle with ageist stereotypes; remember in Chapter 1, we mentioned Robert Wilson's book, *Feminine Forever*, where the goal was to make women attractive again with HRT. We have moved on from those days, but we still need to go further and give women a voice and choice in regard to their sexual health, sexual function, and sexual well-being during and after menopause, and we can start to do that by changing our attitudes to sexuality at midlife by adopting a sex-positive attitude.

Although the roots of sex positivity can be traced back to the feminist movement of the 1960s and 1970s, it's only recently that sex therapists and psychosexual therapists have been pushing for a more sex-positive approach. Sexuality is a vibrant and pleasurable aspect of life that can be embraced at any stage of life, can be an expression of your identity, and should be celebrated. Sex positivity encourages the acceptance and integration of a liberated perspective on sex and sexual pleasure.[13]

Having a sex-positive mindset enables you to explore your sexuality in a healthy and enjoyable way, allowing you to discover and understand what brings you the most pleasure. Embracing a sex-positive attitude involves:

1. **Acceptance and respect**: For your own sexuality and body autonomy. This means choosing to engage in sexual activities because you genuinely want to, not because you feel obligated to do so.
2. **Freedom of choice and sexual desire**: Cultivating a relationship with your own pleasure, body, and body image that is open and non-judgemental.
3. **Compassionate and non-judgemental listening**: Being able to listen to other women talk about their experiences with sex without passing judgement and showing empathy towards their feelings and perspectives.
4. **Open and clear communication**: This involves communicating openly and honestly about sex, boundaries, and desires in a non-judgemental and empathic way.
5. **Respecting personal boundaries**: Both your own and those of your sexual partners.
6. **Honesty about freedom, choices, and preferences**: Encouraging women to have a voice and make choices that align with their own desires and preferences when it comes to experiencing sexual pleasure.

A sex-positive attitude is all about fostering a sense of openness, empowerment, and freedom when it comes to exploring your sexuality. It allows us to embrace our desires, communicate effectively, and prioritise our own pleasure and well-being. By adopting this mindset, women approaching menopause or in the postmenopause stage of life can create more fulfilling and satisfying sexual experiences for themselves and their partners.

TREATMENTS AND SOLUTIONS

Sexual health is integral to our identity and relationships, regardless of our level of engagement. When sexual issues arise, they can significantly impact individuals and relationships with others. If these issues are left unsaid and untreated, they can have serious negative consequences for a couple. That's why placing sexual well-being at the centre of healthcare for women going through and after menopause is essential. Healthcare providers should include a question about any sexual concerns as part of their routine consultation, and they should be familiar with the most common therapeutic techniques to treat their patient's sexual concerns or refer them to specialised psychosexual therapists. Depending on the sexual issue, psychotherapy or psychosexual therapy may be used alone or in conjunction with medical treatments, HRT and non-hormonal medications, and physical therapy (pelvic floor exercises, for example). Even when the sexual issue is primarily biological, CBT works very well.[14] Counselling and psychotherapy (as discussed in chapter one) are useful to explore issues around mood, anxiety, other potential, influential issues and/ or relationship issues.

PSYCHOSEXUAL THERAPY

Psychosexual therapy is a form of counselling and psychotherapy that uses specific techniques to address problems of sexual desire, arousal, orgasm, and pain. It focuses on psychological and sociocultural factors contributing to sexual problems. Interventions generally consist of psychoeducation, couples exercises, and individual and psychotherapeutic approaches.[15] You should never feel self-conscious about asking for professional assistance like this – people of all ages seek help from psychosexual therapists. Popular media often misrepresents sex therapy, suggesting that it involves physical intimacy or hands-on practices. This portrayal is entirely inaccurate. Psychosexual therapy is talking therapy that explores a person's or couple's views, beliefs, attitudes, and behaviours in relation to sex. It's a specialised counselling approach, and any homework or suggestions for intimacy or sexual acts take place in the privacy of a person's or couple's own home and not in the counselling office.

Psychosexual therapy can help with any kind of intimacy difficulty, regardless of whether it is caused by declining hormones, menopause symptoms, medication, or physical or mental health conditions. The psychosexual therapist is not only trained in the therapeutic discipline of counselling but will also have the knowledge of how bodies function and medical conditions that can affect sexual performance, including libido, and will research and be informed on issues of intimacy and sexuality. You can rest assured that there are lots of options available to enhance sexual well-being, regardless of age or menopause.

CONCLUSION

Menopause presents a significant opportunity for women and their healthcare providers to have important discussions and make improvements to their overall health. By addressing physiological changes, symptoms, treatment options, screening recommendations, and psychosocial issues, healthcare providers can contribute to a woman's well-being during the menopause transition and beyond. Over the past few decades, advancements have been made in understanding female sexual function and dysfunction, leading to clearer definitions and models that reflect the lived experiences of women. It can be comforting to know that you're not the only one with these issues, and that there are tried and tested solutions for just about everything. Help is available. However, it is crucial not to treat age-related changes in sexual function as psychologically abnormal and to risk labelling healthy women as dysfunctional. Instead, a comprehensive assessment of various factors and an emphasis on women's satisfaction and well-being can help avoid over-medicalising age-related changes. By addressing all aspects of women's sexual function, researchers and clinicians can better understand and improve this vital component of women's well-being during midlife and beyond.

NOTES

1 Von Hippel et al. (2019).
2 American Psychiatric Association (2013).

3 Thomas et al. (2014).

4 Steckenrider (2023).

5 Erens et al. (2019).

6 Miguel et al. (2024).

7 Steckenrider (2023).

8 Ghizzani (2020).

9 Thomas et al. (2014).

10 Zeanah and Schwarz (1996).

11 Masters and Johnson (1970).

12 Rydberg and Vegunata (2023).

13 Fahs (2014).

14 Spence (2013).

15 Vosper et al. (2021).

6

A LIFE WORTH LIVING – POSITIVE PSYCHOLOGY AND POSITIVE AGEING

INTRODUCTION

Throughout our lifetime, we go through a series of distinct phases, collectively called our life cycle, which has different social and behavioural elements. These phases or stages are shaped by the passage of time as well as significant life milestones, events, and transitions. When it comes to navigating through them, we sometimes find ourselves confronted with loss and the need to adapt to changes in our health, well-being, and roles in society. One typical but significant transition for women is menopause, which is a milestone that can, for some, profoundly affect their overall health and happiness. During and after menopause, women experience a range of physical changes that are closely intertwined with the concept of ageing. For many, menopause is the turning point for acknowledging and accepting that they are getting old, and, like menopause, growing older is an inevitable part of life's journey, presenting us with both challenges and opportunities.

But, for you, the idea of getting older doesn't have to be a daunting prospect because by adopting the right mindset and approach, getting older can be a fulfilling and rewarding journey. It's called positive

DOI: 10.4324/9781003438342-6

ageing, and in this chapter, we will explore that together with the principles from positive psychology that can help you gracefully get through the complexities of ageing. By embracing these principles and incorporating them into your life, you can cultivate resilience, foster meaningful connections, and enhance your overall well-being as you tackle the stages of midlife and postmenopause.

GETTING OLDER, LIVING LONGER

On the bigger stage, the global population is ageing rapidly, and this is presenting multiple challenges for societies worldwide. As we live longer, the proportion of older individuals in our society is steadily increasing, and this is a significant medical and social issue that affects the entire world. According to the World Health Organization, we are generally living longer than previous generations across most parts of the world thanks to a dramatic decline in childhood mortality, advances in medicine, improving living standards, and healthier lifestyles – a welcome development, of course. The life expectancy of humans has doubled in the last century, and the proportion of older people in the population is growing.[1]

This hasn't always been the case – the phenomenon of an ageing population is relatively recent in historical terms. In 1950, no country had more than 11% of its population aged 65 years and older. By 2000, this percentage had increased to a maximum of 18%. However, by 2050, the United Nations (2019) has projected that the problem will escalate significantly with the potential for 38% of the population to be aged 65 years and older.[2] That's double what it is now – a huge change. They also estimate that older women will comprise 54% of the total population by that time, and this idea is often referred to as the feminisation of the population worldwide."[3] It's a very significant statistic as it implies that numerous women will find themselves in the postmenopause stage of life and may have to face age-related health issues. This makes the idea of positive and healthy ageing particularly relevant to anyone reading this book.

According to the World Health Organization, by 2030, one in six people in the world will be aged 60 or over. Between 2015 and 2050, the proportion of the world's population over 60 will almost double, from 12% to 22% the number of people aged 80 years or older is expected to triple between 2020 and 2050 to reach 426 million.

The trend of an ageing population, as noted by the United Nations, is unprecedented and profound and brings significant challenges to all societies. This demographic shift has wide-ranging implications for healthcare, social welfare, labour markets, and economic growth. There are social and psychological ramifications to increased longevity, and while there are obstacles, there are also opportunities, too. If we embrace the idea of an ageing population, we can tackle the challenges by making sure that people not only live longer but also live lives filled with joy, fulfilment, and good health. So, how do we confront these challenges? The United Nations has stepped up to address these issues.

The United Nations *Decade of Healthy Ageing* (2021–2030) is a plan developed by the United Nations General Assembly, and the World Health Organization has been tasked with overseeing its implementation. This initiative aims to address health disparities and enhance the well-being of older individuals, their families, and communities through collective efforts in four key areas:

1. Challenging ageism and promoting positive attitudes towards ageing
2. Creating communities that empower older adults
3. Delivering person-centred integrated care and primary health services tailored to their needs
4. Ensuring access to high-quality long-term care for those who require it

It is interesting to note that during the same period of the United Nations *Decade of Healthy Ageing*, there has been a growing focus on menopause in Western societies. Governments began to prioritise raising awareness about menopause and finding ways to enhance the well-being of women going through this life stage and those who have already experienced it. Menopause and ageing can be seen as interconnected aspects of a woman's life – in other words, meno-pause and ageing are two sides of the same coin. But before we really explore the topic, we need to examine a few interesting facts and figures regarding women during the postmenopausal phase.

MENOPAUSE AND AGEING

As we've seen, the World Health Organization estimates that the proportion of women in the population will continue to increase, with women accounting for 54% of the world. This feminisation of ageing is compounded by the fact that women tend to outlive men in almost every country. In developed nations, women usually live between four and ten years longer than men, while in developing countries, 58% of older adults are women. The significance of this data cannot be overlooked, as it suggests that a large number of women will enter the postmenopausal stage of life, which technically lasts until the end of a woman's life, and there, they may confront age-related health challenges. This underscores the importance of promoting positive and healthy ageing as menopause serves as a reminder of the ageing process. By 2025, they estimate that approximately 1.1 billion living women worldwide will have gone through menopause.[4] According to the United Nations, there were 986 million women aged 50 and above in 2020, and this number is projected to increase to 1.65 billion by 2050. Therefore, most women spend a significant portion of their lives in the postmenopause stage. I should point out here that every woman experiences these changes differently, and there is a wide age range for when they enter the postmenopausal stage.

MENOPAUSAL SYMPTOMS IN POST MENOPAUSE

It is commonly believed that all the troublesome symptoms of menopause disappear once postmenopause begins. Now, this may be true for some women, but others can still experience symptoms similar to those in the perimenopause stage. A study conducted by Lillis and colleagues (2021)[5] found that out of a total of 236 postmenopausal women studied, 59% experienced 13 or more symptoms. The most frequently reported symptoms were hot flushes, affecting 92% of women, low sex drive affecting 89% of women, and night sweats affecting 87% of women. It's important to remember that menopause related symptoms may diminish or disappear altogether after perimenopause, however, some women may still encounter challenges during the postmenopausal stage.

Having a positive attitude towards ageing is extremely important for everyone, particularly women who are going through or have gone through menopause. It helps them to embrace and anticipate a meaningful life beyond this transition. With a positive mindset, women can navigate the journey through menopause and the postmenopausal period with reduced stress and anxiety. In the following section, we will look into the psychological perspective of positive ageing, aiming to fulfil one of the four objectives outlined in the United Nation *Decade of Healthy Ageing* framework. We'll explore how our thoughts, emotions, and behaviours can shape our perception of age and combat ageism. But first, let's look at how positive psychology has contributed to our understanding and management of both our physical and mental well-being.

POSITIVE PSYCHOLOGY AND HEALTH

According to the World Health Organization, health is not just the absence of illness or weakness, but it encompasses a person's overall physical, mental, and social well-being. Although this definition has gained widespread acceptance over the years, the concept of well-being has become so common that it risks losing its true meaning and becoming a cliché. Positive psychology has introduced a new term specifically focused on ageing: positive ageing. This theoretical approach to gerontology (the scientific study of old age) combines disease prevention and wellness to highlight the importance of an individual's mindset in promoting longevity and a high quality of life. Positive psychology is increasingly popular within the broader field of psychology, and research in this area has given us valuable insights into the factors that influence our health and well-being. These advancements have emphasised the significance of personal resources in enhancing our overall wellness. Before we continue, let's clarify the definition and main characteristics of positive psychology.

Positive psychology is a scientific discipline that examines various factors that contribute to a flourishing and thriving life. These factors include experiencing positive emotions, finding purpose and meaning in life, engaging in fulfilling work, and maintaining strong and meaningful relationships. Positive psychologists examine personal strengths, available resources, and positive attributes to understand their impact on our overall well-being. Positive psychology covers a wide range of psychological, social, and societal indicators of our well-being.[6]

Extensive research shows again and again that physical, mental, and social well-being are not only essential aspects of our overall health but are also intricately interconnected with each other. In fact, more and more evidence support the idea that a contented, involved, and satisfying psychological and social existence is not merely a result of good health; it actively contributes to leading us towards a prolonged and healthy life.

The field of psychology has traditionally and successfully focused its efforts on alleviating pain, suffering, and problems. Over time, it has made notable progress in understanding and addressing both physical and mental health concerns. However, the emergence of positive psychology, spearheaded by Martin Seligman in 1998, has expanded our understanding of health beyond just managing it. Positive psychology now encompasses our holistic well-being, aiming to help us to flourish. In doing this, positive psychology emphasises the development of positive attributes at both the individual and group levels. The conventional focus on symptoms and illnesses is undergoing a gradual transformation into a broader understanding of health that encompasses our personal well-being and not just the absence of diseases. Health is now viewed as a valuable asset for everyday living, a positive concept that highlights both social and personal resources in addition to physical capacities.

AGEING AND AGEISM

The increase in life expectancy is, of course, a welcome development. Although an ageing society poses challenges, it also offers numerous opportunities and benefits for older individuals and society as a whole. The primary objective for governments and society at large is to ensure that we can continue to have healthy, happy, and meaningful lives as we live longer. Healthy ageing, also referred to as 'positive ageing' or 'successful ageing,' cannot be achieved through a one-size-fits-all approach. Every individual's journey is distinct and influenced by their specific circumstances, experiences, and aspirations. Positive ageing embraces a comprehensive perspective that acknowledges the multifaceted nature of the ageing process. It involves addressing our evolving physical, emotional, social, spiritual, and cognitive needs as we navigate through our various life stages.

While ageing can bring about many rewarding experiences, it is also a time of significant change. Physical vitality and function may diminish, social networks may shrink, and employment opportunities may become limited. Additionally, the experience of loss, whether it be the loss of loved ones or the loss of certain abilities, can be particularly challenging. But by maintaining a positive attitude towards ageing, we can navigate these changes with confidence and resilience.

Ageing is an inherent aspect of human existence. The way we perceive and handle the ageing process can significantly influence our overall physical and mental health, as well as our understanding and handling of this natural progression. Furthermore, society's outlook towards older people plays a crucial role in shaping our understanding and management of ageing.

Ageism is a critical issue that should not be overlooked. Within Western societies, there exists a prevalent misconception surrounding ageing and older individuals that is rooted in bias, discrimination, and prejudice. These stereotypes depict older adults as dependent, helpless, and lacking value to society due to perceived physical or mental limitations. Research from the Centre for Ageing in the United Kingdom found that that one in three individuals associates older age with frailty, vulnerability, and dependency. When people internalise these cultural biases and prejudices, their self-worth and significance may diminish, leading to feelings of depression and anxiety about the ageing process. In the UK, ageism has been identified as the most widespread form of discrimination, according to research conducted by the Age Without Limits organisation. Alarmingly, half of people aged 50 and over in England have experienced age discrimination within the past year, and half of individuals surveyed express concerns about growing older, with one in five worrying about it frequently.

BLUE ZONES

To shift our perspective on ageing, we need to examine not just the longevity worldwide but also the overall well-being and quality of life experienced by people who live to a ripe old age in good health. We can see that progress in medical and scientific domains, coupled with enhanced healthcare and greater accessibility to health services, has greatly contributed to the extension of our lifespan. While this is generally seen as positive news, there may be concerns about the challenges of ageing and how to maintain both longevity and good health. Is it just an ideal concept or something that can actually be achieved? Recent research by Dan Buettner[7] suggests that living a long and healthy life is not out of reach for us. In fact, he has identified five regions around the world where it is common for people to live well beyond 100 while enjoying happiness, good health, and an active lifestyle. He calls these regions the Blue Zones. Buettner and his team at National Geographic have pinpointed nine key factors that residents in Blue Zones have in common. They include:

1. Regular exercise
2. Plant based diet
3. Having a sense of purpose in life

4. Practicing mindful eating (stopping at 80% fullness)
5. Maintaining a fulfilling social life
6. Alcohol in moderation
7. Maintaining close connections with family and loved one
8. Managing stress effectively – making space for downtime
9. Engaging in community and establishing social support networks

His highly popular publication *The Blue Zones – Secrets for Living Longer* gives us a comprehensive exploration of the principles behind Blue Zones and serves as an inspiring resource to encourage all of us to reflect on and transform our lifestyles to achieve optimal health and well-being.

POSITIVE AGEING

While ageing is often seen as an unavoidable part of life, it does not necessarily mean poor health, decline, or limited mobility. People's health can vary greatly, but there are actions we can take to delay or improve our overall well-being. This is not just wishful thinking or pseudo-empowerment; there is a substantial body of evidence that shows lifestyle and behavioural changes, and personal resources can have a significant and positive impact on our physical and mental health, as well as our brain health. By exploring the principles of positive psychology, we can identify the key personal resources that help us to take control of our health. While we may not be able to change everything, we can focus on the factors we can change and embrace positive and healthy ageing and the privileges it brings.

Positive ageing is about the process of growing older in a way that promotes and maintains a sense of well-being, fulfilment, and purpose. It encompasses a holistic approach to ageing that focuses on maximising physical, emotional, social, and cognitive health as we move to various stages of later life.

Key components of positive ageing include:[8]

Physical health: Positive ageing involves adopting healthy lifestyle behaviours, such as regular exercise, a nutritious diet, adequate sleep, and preventive healthcare measures. Maintaining physical health helps us to remain active and independent as we grow older.

Emotional well-being: With emotional resilience, self-acceptance, and the ability to adapt to life changes. It involves cultivating a positive outlook, managing stress effectively, and engaging in activities that bring joy and fulfilment.

Social connections: Social engagement and support networks play a crucial role in positive ageing. Maintaining meaningful relationships with family, friends, and people in our communities fosters a sense of belonging and provides emotional support during life transitions.

Cognitive function: Keeping the mind active and engaged is essential for positive ageing. Activities such as lifelong learning, cognitive exercises, and creative pursuits help preserve cognitive function and prevent the cognitive decline associated with ageing.

Purpose and meaning: Maintaining a sense of purpose and meaning in life. This may involve pursuing personal goals, engaging in volunteer work or community involvement, and finding activities that provide a sense of fulfilment and contribution.

Adaptation to change: Embracing change and adapting to new circumstances as individuals age. This includes adjusting to retirement, changes in physical health, and transitions in family and social roles.

Resilience: In the face of challenges and adversities associated with ageing. This involves developing coping strategies, seeking support when needed, and maintaining a positive attitude towards age-related changes.

In summary, positive ageing emphasises a proactive and holistic approach to growing older, focusing on maximising well-being, maintaining independence, and embracing the opportunities and challenges that come with ageing. It promotes a positive and empowering perspective on the ageing process, recognising that ageing can be a time of growth, fulfilment, and continued personal development.

CONCLUSION

Overall, positive ageing (as its name implies) emphasises a proactive and holistic approach to growing older, focusing on maximising well-being, maintaining independence, and embracing the opportunities and challenges that come with ageing. The exploration of positive ageing and its potential benefits for women approaching and after menopause has shed light on the transformative power of a positive ageing mindset and behaviours during this important phase of life. The principles derived from positive psychology have illuminated the path to a fulfilling and satisfying ageing process, providing invaluable insights into maintaining overall well-being and navigating the challenges associated with menopause. Throughout this chapter, we have emphasised the potential for growth, self-discovery, and empowerment as women embrace this new stage of life. By incorporating the principles of positive ageing and the strategies we discussed, women can enhance their physical and mental well-being and their brain health, cultivate a sense of purpose, and embark on a journey of personal fulfillment with confidence, resilience, and optimism. Menopause, when viewed through the lens of positive psychology and positive ageing, becomes an opportunity for transformation, self-care, and personal growth. Women can not only weather the challenges of menopause but also thrive, celebrating their wisdom, accomplishments, and continued vitality. We have seen how positive ageing empowers women to embrace the full spectrum of their experiences while living a meaningful, purposeful, and fulfilling life as they approach menopause and beyond. In Chapter 7, the final chapter of this book, we'll see ten evidence-based strategies that can easily become new positive habits to improve your physical and mental wellness and your brain health.

NOTES

1 Bigna et al. (2020).
2 Rudnicka et al. (2020).

3 Mariscal-de-Gante et al. (2023).
4 Shifren and Glass (2014).
5 Lillis et al. (2021).
6 Bolier et al. (2013).
7 Buettner (2022).
8 Robertson (2020).

7

ESTABLISHING AND MAINTAINING WELLNESS DURING AND AFTER MENOPAUSE

INTRODUCTION

Menopause can be the most significant psychological, physiological, and emotional change in a woman's life. It brings with it many physical and psychological challenges and symptoms and can have a serious impact on brain health. There are, however, a number of self-care strategies every woman can implement to help get them through their change of life. It's not just about coping with the changes and their effects, but it's also about improving your quality of life both now and for the rest of your life.

In this chapter, we will explore the different self-care techniques you can use and how important they are to your well-being. Hopefully, I can arm you with the tools you need to manage the symptoms of menopause and embrace the change of life with resilience, hope, and energy. We will take a look at neuroscience research and, in particular, the concept of neuroplasticity, which is the brain's remarkable ability to reorganize itself and adapt to new experiences. By understanding the physiology of your brain to form new neural connections, you can

DOI: 10.4324/9781003438342-7

understand how the phenomenon can help you to form new habits and change your behaviour in a positive way. We will discuss the psychology of habits and help you to make positive changes during menopause by adopting positive health habits.

We'll look at ten self-care strategies that can help you clear the brain fog, as it's called, improve your mood, enhance your physical well-being, and get more and better sleep. With these practical tools, I hope to help you navigate the transitions of menopause and reach your best health. We'll look at evidence-based approaches that will help you embrace this important stage of your life with strength, confidence, and positivity.

WHAT IS SELF-CARE?

Self-care is obviously about you taking care of yourself. It's about tending to your physical and emotional needs and being the best person physically and emotionally that you can be. Self-care is not self-indulgent or being self-centred; it's about taking deliberate actions to nurture yourself and improve your physical, emotional, and mental health.

For many women going through menopause, life can be particularly challenging as they try to balance the demands of family, work, ageing parents, and childcare. Is it any wonder that stress levels can go through the roof? Burnout and even breakdown can be real possibilities, which is why you should take care of yourself using self-care techniques to boost your resilience and balance in life.

All over the world, there is a growth in self-care practises, which shows that more and more people everywhere recognise the significance of their own responsibility for their own well-being and mental health. Recent data and research shows that self-care practises have quadrupled in popularity since 2018, and more and more people are looking to incorporate these strategies into their daily routines.

Self-care is not a selfish act. Always remember that we're talking about you taking care of yourself so that you can take care of your life and of everyone else that you need to look after. Make self-care a priority.[1]

Please remember that using self-care practises on their own may not bring all the answers you're looking for: you need to get lots of high-quality sleep, for example. If you get a lot of exercise, that's great. But you also need a well-balanced and nutrient-rich diet. If you've got everything else working well for you, but you're not getting enough water, you could be in trouble, too. What you need to do is take an integrated, holistic approach to your self-care. This kind of planning and multifaceted care will not only help you get through menopause but also improve your quality of life thereafter. You can create new and positive habits that become a part of your life, you need to be resolute, focused, and determined to make small changes every day.

Research has shown that a person's attitude is a stronger predictor of their behaviour than their intentions are. In other words, we may have the best intentions in the world, but we may not succeed in taking good care of ourselves. Having a positive attitude and taking personal responsibility and control of the things you can control is far more effective in helping maintain stronger physical, mental, and brain health.

Make sure you put aside time for yourself and engage in deliberate behaviours that will create positive health habits and self-care practises. If you do this, you're not only going to create new helpful habits you will also develop a toolkit for self-care activities that will support you throughout your journey to menopause and beyond. Make a commitment to yourself to make it a healthy transition through this potentially difficult time.

SELF-CARE FOR MENOPAUSE

Self-care is particularly important for pre and postmenopausal women, who often face unique challenges during these two phases. Hormone levels can fluctuate wildly, and the resulting emotional issues can take a heavy toll on your physical and mental health. This is why your new self-care practices should be tailored to address these specific needs. Self-care routines that focus on hormone regulation, emotional support, physical well-being, and sleep quality will help you to get through those changes more effectively and improve your overall quality of life. For example, practicing meditation to manage stress levels or prioritising sleep hygiene to support hormone balance can make a huge difference with both of these issues.

Self-care does not have to be costly or extravagant. You can integrate it seamlessly into your daily routines without spending any money whatsoever. By incorporating self-care practises into your everyday life, such as spending time in nature or practising gratitude, you can use zero-cost tools that significantly benefit your well-being. They not only promote relaxation and stress relief but also foster mindfulness and a sense of presence in our day-to-day lives. Self-care is accessible to absolutely everyone and can be tailored to suit your own personal preferences and needs.

NEUROPLASTICITY

In Chapter 3, we explored the concept of neuroplasticity, which is about the brain's remarkable ability to alter its structure and function in response to experiences, thoughts, and emotions. This is crucial for brain development and learning, as it involves the formation of new neural connections, the strengthening of existing ones, and the elimination of unused ones.

Thanks to advancements in neuroscience research, particularly in imaging technologies, scientists have made groundbreaking discoveries about the ever-changing nature of our brains throughout our lives. This debunks the long-held belief that our brains are fixed and unchangeable after a certain age. While the rate of change may change as we grow older, our brains possess an incredible capacity for dynamic growth and adaptation.[2]

Knowing this should bring us great comfort when it comes to enhancing our health and well-being. Now we can be confident about learning new behaviours and adopting fresh perspectives, not only to improve our well-being, but also to support optimal brain health during and after menopause.

THE PSYCHOLOGY OF HABITS

Our lives are driven by habits – actions and behaviours that, through repetition, become automatic and routine. Building positive habits can have a remarkable impact on both our physical and mental well-being, and to understand how we can create and maintain these positive habits, we must first explore the psychology behind them. Neuroscience research shows us that habits are comprised of three key factors, referred to as the habit loop: cue, routine, and reward. Ok, so let's look at each one in detail.[3]

THE HABIT LOOP: CUE, ROUTINE, AND REWARD

Cue: The cue is a trigger that initiates a specific habit. It can be something in our environment, a specific time of day, or even an emotional state. For example, the smell of brewing coffee may trigger the desire to get a cup of coffee.

Routine: The routine is the habit itself or the action that we automatically perform in response to the cue. In our example, the routine might be walking to the coffee maker and pouring a cup.

Reward: The reward is the positive outcome we experience because of performing the routine, which reinforces the habit loop. In the case of coffee, the reward might be the pleasant taste and the increased alertness we feel after drinking a cup.

ATOMIC HABITS

Understanding the habit loop is crucial to building positive habits because it helps us to identify the cues and rewards we need to control in order to encourage good habits. According to James Clear, author of the best-selling book *Atomic Habits*, the key to creating effective, automatic habits lies in making them obvious, attractive, easy, and satisfying.

Obvious: Make the cues for your habit obvious and available in your daily routine so that you are consistently reminded of the habit.

Attractive: Make the habit appealing so that you are motivated to follow through and continue the routine.

Easy: Remove any barriers to performing the habit so that it is simple and easily done.

Satisfying: Ensure that the habit provides immediate satisfaction, which will solidify the habit loop and reinforce habit formation.

Crafting practical steps for lasting positive habits

To create and sustain lasting positive habits, try including the following steps in your daily routine:

Identify the habit loop: Reflect on the actions that you want to transform into habits and break them down into cues, routines, and rewards.

Make the habit obvious: Design your environment to support the habit you want to develop. Place visual reminders and triggers in easily seen locations, helping make the habit hard to ignore.

Set achievable goals: Start small and gradually increase the habit's difficulty as you build momentum.

Track your progress: Keep track of your progress to stay motivated and increase the satisfaction of maintaining a positive habit.

Stay committed: Remember that habits take time to form, so be patient.

By accepting that habits influence our actions, we can use neuroplasticity to rewire our brains positively. That's huge. This understanding means that we can intentionally shape our environment and daily routines to cultivate the positive habits we want in our lives. Through consistent and deliberate practice and taking advantage of the brain's neuroplasticity, we can make long-lasting changes that will help improve our overall well-being. But please be patient and remember that habits and routines take time to become a part of our lives. James Clear also emphasises the importance of adopting a 'never miss twice' mindset, which acts as a powerful tool for overcoming setbacks or lapses. It revolves around understanding that it's ok to slip and have lapses occasionally, but it's very important not to let one slip completely derail your progress.[4]

TEN SELF-CARE STRATEGIES

Here are ten practical self-care practises tailored specifically for menopausal women to help them navigate this transition with strength and energy. By embracing these strategies as positive habits for your overall well-being, they can easily be integrated into your daily or weekly routine. The goal is to use self-care practises so that they become an integral part of your life, as effortless and automatic habits, promoting resilience and vitality during this transformative phase.

1. BOOST BRAIN HEALTH

Given our focus on the complexities of the brain and its incredible ability to support our functioning, it is only appropriate that we begin our ten strategies with improving brain health and safeguarding its well-being. We'll also explore strategies to overcome the challenges presented by brain fog.

In chapter three, we looked at the phenomenon of brain fog, which can be experienced by many women during menopause. Although not a condition or a syndrome, brain fog relates to feeling muddled and confused and finding it difficult to concentrate. Brain fog can have various causes, including hormonal fluctuations and illness, and it can manifest as difficulties in memory recall, forgetting people's names, and an inability to focus. The good news is that research has identified strategies that can help alleviate it, so let's consider some beneficial habits we can develop. Bear in mind that while it may not be entirely possible to prevent menopause-related brain fog completely, there are some lifestyle changes you can make to potentially mitigate symptoms and improve your overall memory.[5]

HOW TO BEAT BRAIN FOG

- Pay attention to your diet and reduce sugar, caffeine, and alcohol.
- Get lots of quality sleep – the brain cannot function effectively without enough good quality sleep.
- Manage stress levels – stress in small doses can actually be good for us as it keeps us motivated and is good for learning. When adrenaline levels are high, your brain and body are alert and aware, ready to jump into action. A neuromodulator called acetylcholine, which is involved in sharpening your focus and helping you to filter out unnecessary information rises too. As you become focused on your work, you get a dopamine hit – which is the 'feel good' neurotransmitter. However, short-term stress can become chronic stress if you don't learn how to manage it (see Chapter 3 for more about stress and how to manage it).
- Speak to your healthcare provider about checking to see if you have adequate levels of vitamin B12, vitamin D, and omega 3. These vitamins are essential nutrients for your brain functioning.
- Take up some mentally stimulating activities, learn something new, and start a new hobby – midlife is a time when you have more free time, so take advantage of that and learn a new language. Continue learning new skills throughout your lifetime to give your brain a regular workout.
- Limit or avoid multitasking – focus on one task at a time.
- Get daily exercise and aim for a good life/work balance.

In summary, adopting a well-balanced diet, ensuring adequate sleep, and engaging in regular exercise are commonly recommended practises for promoting overall good health. These habits contribute to physical and psychological well-being and brain health.

2. PRACTICE SELF-COMPASSION

Menopause can be overwhelming. When faced with the symptoms of menopause plus the pressures of life, it can be easy to neglect your own well-being. We set lofty goals for ourselves, and while we want to be perfect, sometimes we criticise ourselves when we don't feel we have reached our own visions of who and what we should be. Research shows that practising self-compassion can have a significant positive impact on her mental health, resilience, and relationships.[6] Don't forget that even small changes can lead to big changes over time. Now let's try to understand what self-compassion really means.

Self-compassion, as the name suggests, is about showing yourself kindness, acceptance, and compassion during difficult times. Recognise the pain that judgement brings and treat yourself with the same level of care and love that you offer other loved ones. A lot of research has shown that this can have a profound effect on our overall well-being.

One of the biggest benefits is a positive effect on her mental well-being. When you cultivate self-compassion, you can reduce negative thoughts and emotions. Then, you can acknowledge the pain without the harsh self-criticism that can sometimes go with it. As a result, we experience lower levels of anxiety, depression, and stress, which leads to improved emotional well-being.

Self-compassion can also build your resilience. When you are kind and understanding towards yourself, you increase your ability to bounce back from setbacks and face challenges with greater strength and determination. Self-compassion can help create a solid base for personal growth and empowerment.

Practising self-compassion is essential for our overall well-being. It not only improves our mental health by reducing negative thoughts and emotions, but it also enhances our resilience in the face of adversity. By treating ourselves with kindness and understanding, we can cultivate a sense of inner strength and compassion that positively impacts our relationships and our ability to navigate life's challenges. So, make a conscious effort to prioritise self-compassion and experience the transformative power it brings.

HOW TO PRACTICE SELF-COMPASSION

- Treat yourself with kindness and respect like you would a good friend.
- Nurture your body with healthy eating, daily exercise, and rest.
- Silence the inner critic – replace self-criticism with positive self-talk. Forgive yourself for mistakes, past or present.
- Focus on your character strengths and personal resources – your best qualities.
- Practice mindfulness and meditation to be aware of your feelings and thoughts.
- Any one, or all, of these ten strategies will help you to tap into your self-compassion by prioritising self-care.

3. PRACTICE GRATITUDE

Expressing gratitude is a powerful emotion that has a profound effect on our well-being. It involves acknowledging and valuing the positive elements in life – the ones that bring us joy and fulfilment. Countless studies have shown the positive effects of gratitude on overall well-being. For example, research conducted by Emmons and Stern (2013)[7] revealed that people who regularly practice gratitude have elevated levels of happiness, optimism, and life satisfaction. They also experience fewer signs of depression and stress.

Gratitude plays a significant role in improving mental health by redirecting our focus away from negative thoughts and emotions. It helps us shift our attention towards the positive aspects of our lives, nurturing a sense of contentment and fulfilment. Through the practice of gratitude, individuals cultivate a more optimistic perspective, which can act as a buffer against stress and promote resilience.

HOW TO PRACTICE GRATITUDE

- Say a spontaneous thank you to someone who has, unbeknownst to them, been kind to you or helped you with something.
- Share the good feelings you felt from someone's kindness with that person.
- Keep a gratitude journal, reflect on all the things you are grateful for, and appreciate each moment of every day.

Practising gratitude is a really fulfilling practice and can help you to build an appreciation for both the current moment and past experiences. Research from Morin (2014)[8] found that thanking a new acquaintance makes them more likely to seek a more lasting relationship with you. People who show gratitude report fewer aches and pains, a general feeling of healthiness, take more exercise, enjoy higher levels of well-being and happiness, and suffer less from symptoms of depression.

Multiple studies show us that engaging in gratitude leads to increased levels of happiness, optimism, and overall satisfaction with life. Simultaneously, it reduces symptoms of depression and stress.

4. IMPROVE SLEEP QUALITY AND DURATION

Have you heard of 'sleep hygiene'? It's about practicing a 'clean' path to getting a really good, restful, refreshing sleep at night. It encompasses a range of practises and behaviours that are crucial for achieving a good rest at the end of the day and maintaining daytime alertness and vitality. It involves several things, both behavioural and environmental, that can impact the quality of our sleep. If you adopt proper sleep hygiene, you can enhance your sleep quality and overall well-being. Wouldn't that be great? These practises can really improve the quality of our sleep and, so, our overall health. Here are some top tips for promoting good sleep hygiene:[9]

1. **Establish a consistent sleep schedule:** Try to go to bed and wake up at the same time every day, even on weekends or days off. This helps regulate your body's internal clock and promotes a more consistent sleep pattern as your body expects to fall asleep at the same time.
2. **Create a relaxing bedtime routine:** Develop a pre-sleep routine that helps you wind down and signals to your body that it is time to sleep. This may include activities like reading a book, taking a warm bath, or practising relaxation techniques.
3. **Create a sleep-friendly environment:** Make sure your bedroom is quiet, dark, and cool. Use curtains or blinds to block out excess light, earplugs, or white noise machines to minimise noise disturbances. Think about switching to a comfortable mattress and pillows that support your sleeping position.
4. **Limit exposure to screens before bed:** This can be a tough habit to break, but the blue light emitted by electronic devices such as smartphones, tablets, and computers can disrupt your sleep-wake cycle. Avoid using these devices at least an hour before bed to allow your brain to relax and prepare for sleep.
5. **Avoid stimulants and heavy meals before bed**: Caffeine, nicotine, and alcohol can interfere with your ability to fall asleep and stay asleep throughout the night. Additionally, eating a heavy meal close to bedtime can cause discomfort and disrupt your sleep.
6. **Engage in regular physical activity:** Regular exercise during the day can promote better sleep at night. However, avoid exercising too close to bedtime as it may stimulate your body and make it harder to fall asleep.
7. **Manage stress:** High levels of stress can make it difficult to relax and fall asleep. Find healthy ways to manage stress, such as relaxation techniques, hobbies, or support from friends, family, or professional therapists.

Add these practises to your daily routine, and you can significantly improve the quality of the sleep you get at night. Good sleep will improve your overall well-being, which is really important during menopause as it combats some of the challenges and difficulties this stage of life can bring to women. Good sleep hygiene is an ongoing process that needs consistency and commitment from you. If sleep hygiene is not enough for you to get a good night's sleep, talk to your doctor or healthcare professional about sleeping tablets or cognitive behavioural therapy for insomnia (CBTi), which has proven to be very effective.[10]

5. APPRECIATE THE GIFT OF NATURE ON YOUR PHYSICAL, MENTAL, AND BRAIN HEALTH

Nature is good for you. No surprise there. Immersing yourself in the natural world amidst the beauty of nature in green spaces or walking and looking at the sea or a lake view (blue spaces) brings a wide range of benefits for your mental, physical, and brain health.[11]

Here's what nature does for us:

- Numerous studies have revealed that spending time in green spaces can enhance mental well-being, reduce stress levels, lower blood pressure, and alleviate symptoms of depression and anxiety. Simply being exposed to green environments can diminish stress and promote relaxation. Natural surroundings give us a much-needed escape from the demands and pressures of everyday life.
- Spending time outdoors is an excellent way to lift your mood and has a profound positive impact on mental health and overall well-being. You'll also soak up natural sunlight which boosts vitamin D levels crucial for healthy bones and a strong immune system.
- Research has also shown that being in outdoor settings can improve both the duration and quality of your sleep. It is particularly beneficial for women going through menopause and can help

them battle with brain fog by enhancing cognitive function and performance.

- By spending more time in nature, you can gain a heightened sense of happiness and overall life satisfaction. That's because you'll create a deep connection to the natural world and gain a sense of harmony with your surroundings, which brings solace and tranquility in today's fast-paced world.

By immersing ourselves in nature, we not only reap the benefits for our physical and mental health, but we also nurture our brain health and functioning. The healing power of nature is undeniable, offering respite from stress, improving mood, supporting cognitive function, and fostering a profound sense of happiness and connectedness. So, take a step outside every day and let nature work its wonders on your mind and body.

6. ADOPT THE DAILY THE THREE GOOD THINGS EXERCISE

The Three Good Things exercise in positive psychology is a simple but powerful technique that promotes gratitude. You simply think about three positive events or experiences from your day and appreciate the reasons for them happening and the impact they had on you. This practice has been shown to improve mental health. Participants who completed the exercise for a week reported an increased sense of happiness and reduced symptoms of depression, with effects lasting for six months. By focusing on positive experiences every day, this exercise cultivates a grateful mindset and enhances happiness and life satisfaction.[12]

HOW TO DO THE THREE GOOD THINGS EXERCISE

- At the end of every day, make a list of three good things that happened that day.
- Reflect and write down how the three things made you feel.

7. PRACTICE MINDFULNESS

Mindfulness is all about being fully present in the moment, without judgement. It involves being aware of your thoughts, feelings, sensations, and environment to get a deeper understanding of ourselves and our experiences.

Regular mindfulness has many benefits for our well-being. Research shows it can reduce stress by focusing on the present moment without judgement, promoting relaxation and calm. It also improves concentration and productivity, and we know from several studies that regular mindfulness practice has numerous benefits for well-being. It can reduce symptoms of anxiety and depression, and it also helps to improve cognitive function, focus, attention, and emotional regulation.[13]

Self-awareness is key to mindfulness. By being aware of our own thoughts, emotions, and bodily sensations, without judgement, we gain insight into our inner experience. This helps us understand our thinking patterns and behaviours, enabling us to make conscious choices to help reach our goals.

Mindfulness promotes happiness and contentment by focusing on the present moment and letting go of past regrets and future worries. This cultivates gratitude, compassion, and a positive outlook, leading to increased well-being and life satisfaction.

Incorporating mindfulness into your daily life can be done using some or all of these ways:

- **Start with short sessions**: Begin by setting aside a few minutes each day to sit in a quiet space and focus on your breath. Gradually increase the duration of your mindfulness sessions as you become more comfortable.
- Use reminders throughout the day to bring yourself back to the present moment. It can be as simple as a gentle alarm, a sticky note in a visible location, or an app on your phone.
- **Engage in mindful activities:** incorporate mindfulness into activities like walking, eating, or even doing routine household

tasks. Pay attention to the sensations and sounds associated with these activities and fully immerse yourself in the present moment.

8. DEVELOP A POSITIVE MINDSET – DISCOVER THE POWER OF YET

There is mounting evidence that an individual's mindset plays a significant role in their behaviour, as well as their personal and professional lives. By 'mindset,' we mean a mental framework or perspective that guides people in how they interpret experiences and directs their corresponding actions and responses. Interestingly, a single three-letter word, 'yet,' holds the power to instill a growth mindset.

Carole Dweck, a renowned psychologist in the United States, has extensively studied two types of mindsets: fixed and growth. She says that people with a fixed mindset see talent and ability as inherent qualities that they either possess or lack. They believe that skills and knowledge are stable and unchangeable. On the other hand, those with a growth mindset believe that they can develop their abilities through dedication and hard work. They view their brains and talents as mere starting points. This perspective fosters a love for learning and cultivates the resilience needed to achieve success.[14]

People who adopt a growth mindset – the belief that they can learn more or become smarter by exerting effort and persevering – acquire more knowledge more quickly. Embracing a growth mindset encourages us to see challenges as opportunities for personal growth and skill development. This helps some people to take on new challenges, knowing that they have the capacity to enhance their abilities through determined effort.

And when these people make a mistake or encounter unexpected difficulties, they see it as an opportunity for growth rather than becoming discouraged or giving up. People with a growth mindset have the capacity to enhance and broaden their knowledge, skills, and achievements.

All of us can benefit from incorporating the word 'yet' into our daily lives and internal dialogue. Here are a few examples of how this small word can transform a sentence and alter our perspective for the better:

HOW TO USE THE POWER OF YET

- "I can't do this yet."
- "I don't understand this yet."
- "I don't get it yet."
- "I'm not ready yet."
- "I haven't passed the exam yet."
- "I haven't learned this skill set yet."
- "I can't cope with this yet."

Remember that small changes can have big consequences: Research tells us that brief interventions can have lasting effects.

9. TAKE TIME TO RECOGNISE AND JOURNAL YOUR THOUGHTS AND FEELINGS

This might sound strange but think of menopause as a golden opportunity to reflect on your life choices, reassess social and family roles, and embrace a newfound freedom to explore other interests or careers. One way to make the most of this transitional period is by developing the habit of keeping a reflective journal. There is lots and lots of research that supports the numerous benefits of journaling. It promotes self-awareness, provides an outlet for releasing complex emotions, and aids in coping with challenging feelings. Writing and wellness go hand-in-hand, especially when approached with purpose and intention. Journal writing can serve as a powerful tool for healing and personal transformation.

Expressing your thoughts and emotions in a journal fosters insight, self-compassion, and body awareness. It allows you to organise your thoughts and regulate your emotions. Pioneering research by Pennebaker proves that journaling about unpleasant experiences can lead to reduced blood pressure and improved moods. Also, journaling about meaningful topics enhances both physical and emotional well-being, irrespective of personality, culture, or language.[15]

Ultimately, journaling has been proven time and time again to be a means for self-understanding, self-guidance, and fostering expanded creativity.

HOW CAN I BEGIN MY JOURNALING JOURNEY?

- Start by selecting a journal that physically resonates with you – consider the colour, texture, size, and any other preferences you may have.
- Find and stick to a safe and private space where you can reflect on your personal thoughts, document daily events, and explore your evolving insights.
- Giving your thoughts a voice through writing helps you release emotions and gain clarity in the face of complex life experiences. Make sure that you have a secure place to store your journal so that you're never worried about others reading it. Your journal will be a sanctuary for recording your innermost thoughts and emotions, providing a space where you can freely express yourself without fear of judgement, criticism, or analysis. It's an empowering form of self-expression.

In essence, journaling is all about recording your thoughts, perceptions, and emotions. It's about self-expression and self-discovery during the menopausal journey. It's going to help you to navigate your emotions more effectively, gain a deeper understanding of yourself, and experience positive changes in your overall well-being. So, grab a pen and a notebook and embark on this transformative journey of self-reflection.

10. BUILD CONNECTIONS – THE BENEFITS OF SOCIAL SUPPORT

We are social animals, and we need people around us. Ok, not all the time. But social support plays a crucial role in our health, as shown by extensive research that has highlighted its positive impact on both our physical and mental well-being. Studies have consistently demonstrated that social support is a key factor in alleviating menopausal symptoms and enhancing the overall quality of life for women going through it.[16] As women try to navigate the complexities of menopause and make sense of its various symptoms, they often turn to others for guidance and reassurance. Whether it's discussing hot flushes or sharing experiences of mood swings, women find comfort and encouragement in the empathetic and caring demeanour of their friends and family members.

Here are some of the different ways social support can help:

Emotional support: As women experience emotional ups and downs, thanks to hormonal changes and symptoms like mood swings, anxiety, and depression, a supportive network of friends, family, or support groups can give you emotional validation, understanding, and comfort during this time.

Practical support: Social support can also involve practical help with daily tasks or responsibilities that may become more challenging during menopause, especially if women are experiencing symptoms like fatigue or brain fog.

Information and education: Supportive social networks can provide valuable information and education about menopause, including its physical and emotional symptoms, treatment options, lifestyle modifications, and coping strategies. Access to accurate information can empower women to make informed decisions about their health and well-being.

Validation of experiences: Menopause is a totally natural and completely normal part of a woman's life, but it can sometimes be accompanied by feelings of isolation and inadequacy. Social support networks can validate women's experiences and reassure them that they are not alone in their struggles. Sharing experiences with other women going through menopause can help normalise the process and reduce feelings of stigma or, believe it or not, shame.

Encouragement for self-care: Menopause often prompts women to prioritise self-care practises that support their physical and emotional well-being. Social support networks can encourage and reinforce these self-care behaviours, such as getting regular exercise, healthy eating, adequate sleep, stress management, and seeking medical care if it's needed.

Reduced stress and improved coping: Social support can act as a buffer against stress and help women develop effective coping strategies for managing menopausal symptoms and related challenges. Having someone to talk to, seek advice from, or simply share a laugh with can alleviate stress and improve overall resilience during menopause.

Enhanced sense of belonging: Menopause can sometimes lead to changes in social roles and relationships, such as empty nest syndrome or shifts in relationships with your spouse. Social networks provide a sense of belonging and connection, fostering meaningful relationships and a sense of community that can help women navigate these changes more easily.

Ways to seek out support include:

- **Engaging in conversations with loved ones**: Start by reaching out to trusted friends and family members – people you feel comfortable sharing with. Tell them about your experiences, worries, and emotions about menopause. Sometimes, simply discussing your journey can bring about emotional relief and a sense of support.

- **Join support groups:** Consider joining a menopause support group, whether in-person or online. These groups offer a secure and empathetic environment where women who are going through similar experiences can share advice and strategies for coping and give support. Online forums and social media groups that focus on menopause can also be very valuable.
- **Consulting healthcare professionals:** Talk to your doctor about your menopausal symptoms and concerns. They can provide medical guidance, discuss treatment options and refer you to support services such as counselling, therapy, or specialised menopause clinics if you need them. Don't hesitate to ask questions and advocate for your own healthcare needs.
- **Consider counselling or psychological therapy:** Individual or group counselling with a therapist who specialises in women's health or menopause can help you get over the emotional hurdles of menopause, address any pre-existing psychological issues and cultivate practical coping mechanisms. They offer support and guidance and can help you gain insight into your emotions and experiences during menopause, as well as helping you develop strategies to manage them.
- **Explore online resources:** Take the initiative to explore online resources and find reliable information. There are numerous dedicated online resources that provide education, support, and a sense of community for menopause. These resources include websites, blogs, forums, and social media platforms that focus specifically on menopause. They often have a wealth of information, expert advice, and support from others who are going through similar experiences.
- **Attend workshops or educational events:** Consider going to workshops, seminars, or educational events either in your local community or online that focus on topics related to menopause. These events often feature healthcare professionals, and support groups who can provide valuable information, resources, and opportunities for networking.

It is important to remember that seeking social support during menopause is absolutely the right thing to do. You're taking a proactive step towards taking care of your physical, emotional, and mental well-being, so don't hesitate to reach out to others and explore different support options.

CONCLUSION

Embracing change during menopause is a profound journey that calls for resilience, self-compassion, and a proactive approach to holistic well-being. We have explored the pivotal role of self-care in navigating this transformative phase of your life with strength and vitality. We've also shown you the significance of cultivating positive health habits, fostering resilience, and embracing change as an opportunity for growth and self-discovery.

The chapter has shown how important self-care practices are in enhancing physical and psychological well-being during menopause. We have explored the transformative power of self-care, emphasising its role in creating positive health habits that transcend menopausal challenges and contribute to your overall well-being. Understanding the significance of self-care in regulating hormones, promoting emotional balance, and improving the quality of your sleep has been a cornerstone of our exploration.

We have also looked at ten practical self-care practises that can enhance well-being during menopause. From fostering physical well-being through improving sleep to nurturing a positive mindset and harnessing the restorative benefits of nature, these tools can help make menopause a little more manageable for women. Additionally, we've seen the very important therapeutic benefits of social support and community connections, emphasising the transformative impact of building a strong support network and engaging in meaningful relationships.

As we embark on the journey of change menopause brings, it's really important to embrace self-care, which can help you to get through this change of life with resilience and confidence. By integrating these self-care practices into daily life, you can foster a sense of empowerment and mastery. For further information on each of the ten self-care practices, please see page 126. The takeaway message from this Chapter is to prioritise self-care practises that will help you have a positive menopause experience.

NOTES

1 Ferguson et al. (2024).
2 Cramer et al. (2011).
3 Wood and Rünger (2016).
4 Clear (2018).
5 Mosconi (2024).
6 Kynaston (2019).
7 Emmons and Stern (2013).
8 Morin (2014).
9 Irish et al. (2015).
10 Baglioni et al. (2022).
11 Williams (2017).
12 Bolier et al. (2013).
13 Brockman et al. (2016).
14 Dweck (2012).
15 Sohal et al. (2022).
16 Edwards et al. (2021).

REFERENCES

American Psychiatric Association. (2013). *Diagnostic and statistical manual of mental disorders, DSM-5(TM)* (5th ed.). American Psychiatric Publishing.

Antonovsky, A. (2002). *Unraveling the mystery of health: How people manage stress and stay well eBooks* (pp. 127–139). SAGE Publications Ltd. https://doi.org/10.4135/9781446221129.n9

Arnould, A., Rochat, L., Azouvi, P., & Van Der Linden, M. (2013). A multidimensional approach to apathy after traumatic brain injury. *Neuropsychology Review, 23*(3), 210–233. https://doi.org/10.1007/s11065-013-9236-3

Baglioni, C., Espie, C. A., & Riemann, D. (2022). *Cognitive-behavioural therapy for insomnia (CBT-I) across the life span: Guidelines and clinical protocols for health professionals.* John Wiley & Sons.

Bezzant, N. (2022). *This changes everything: The honest guide to menopause and perimenopause.* Penguin Books.

Bigna, J. J., Ndoadoumgue, A. L., Nansseu, J. R., Tochie, J. N., Nyaga, U. F., Nkeck, J. R., Foka, A. J., Kaze, A. D., & Noubiap, J. J. (2020). Global burden of hypertension among people living with HIV in the era of increased life expectancy: A systematic review and meta-analysis. *Journal of Hypertension, 38*(9), 1659–1668. https://doi.org/10.1097/hjh.0000000000002446

Bolier, L., Haverman, M., Westerhof, G. J., Riper, H., Smit, F., & Bohlmeijer, E. (2013). Positive psychology interventions: A meta-analysis of randomized controlled studies. *BMC Public Health, 13*(1). https://doi.org/10.1186/1471-2458-13-119

Bolton, D., & Gillett, G. (2019). *The biopsychosocial model of health and disease: New philosophical and scientific developments*. Springer.

Brockman, R., Ciarrochi, J., Parker, P., & Kashdan, T. (2016). Emotion regulation strategies in daily life: Mindfulness, cognitive reappraisal and emotion suppression. *Cognitive Behaviour Therapy*, 46(2), 91–113. https://doi.org/10.1080/16506073.2016.1218926

Buettner, D. (2022). *The blue zones challenge: A 4-week plan for a longer, better life*. Disney Electronic Content.

Clear, J. (2018). *Atomic habits: An easy & proven way to build good habits & break bad ones*. https://catalog.umj.ac.id/index.php?p=show_detail&id=62390

Cramer, S. C., Sur, M., Dobkin, B. H., O'Brien, C., Sanger, T. D., Trojanowski, J. Q., Rumsey, J. M., Hicks, R., Cameron, J., Chen, D., Chen, W. G., Cohen, L. G., deCharms, C., Duffy, C. J., Eden, G. F., Fetz, E. E., Filart, R., Freund, M., Grant, S. J., & Vinogradov, S. (2011). Harnessing neuroplasticity for clinical applications. *Brain*, 134(6), 1591–1609. https://doi.org/10.1093/brain/awr039

Dignam, L. (2021). *The menopause hub*. www.themenopausehub.ie/menopause-in-the-workplace.

Dweck, C. (2012). *Mindset*. Robinson.

Edwards, A. L., Shaw, P. A., Halton, C. C., Bailey, S. C., Wolf, M. S., Andrews, E. N., & Cartwright, T. (2021). "It just makes me feel a little less alone": A qualitative exploration of the podcast menopause: Unmuted on women's perceptions of menopause. *Menopause*, 28(12), 1374–1384. https://doi.org/10.1097/gme.0000000000001855

Emmons, R. A., & Stern, R. (2013). Gratitude as a psychotherapeutic intervention. *Journal of Clinical Psychology*, 69(8), 846–855. https://doi.org/10.1002/jclp.22020

Erens, B., Mitchell, K. R., Gibson, L., Datta, J., Lewis, R., Field, N., & Wellings, K. (2019). Health status, sexual activity and satisfaction among older people in Britain: A mixed methods study. *PLoS One*, 14(3), e0213835. https://doi.org/10.1371/journal.pone.0213835

Fahs, B. (2014). "Freedom to" and "freedom from": A new vision for sex-positive politics. *Sexualities*, 17(3), 267–290. https://doi.org/10.1177/1363460713516334

Ferguson, L., Anderson, M. E., Satchi, K., Capron, A. M., Kaplan, C. D., Redfield, P., & Gruskin, S. (2024). The ubiquity of 'self-care' in health: Why specificity matters. *Global Public Health*, 19(1). https://doi.org/10.1080/17441692.2023.2296970.

Foxcroft, L. (2010). *Hot flushes, cold science: A history of the modern menopause.* Granta Books.

Freeman, E. W., Sammel, M. D., Liu, L., Gracia, C. R., Nelson, D. B., & Hollander, L. (2004). Hormones and menopausal status as predictors of depression in women in transition to Menopause. *Archives of General Psychiatry, 61*(1), 62. https://doi.org/10.1001/archpsyc.61.1.62

Froman, W. J. (2000). Merleau-Ponty and phenomenological philosophy. *Etudes Phénoménologiques,* 16(31), 83–101. https://doi.org/10.5840/etudphen 20001631/324

Geraghty, P. (2021). *Each woman's menopause: An evidence-based resource: For nurse practitioners, advanced practice nurses and allied health professionals.* Springer Nature.

Ghizzani, A. (2020). *Healthy aging: Well-being and sexuality at menopause and beyond.* Novum Publishing.

Hickey, M., LaCroix, A. Z., Doust, J., Mishra, G. D., Sivakami, M., Garlick, D., & Hunter, M. S. (2024). An empowerment model for managing menopause. *Lancet, 403*(10430), 947–957. https://doi.org/10.1016/s0140-6736(23) 02799-x

Hunter, M., & Smith, M. (2024). *Living well through the menopause: An evidence-based cognitive behavioural guide.* Hachette UK.

Hunter, M. S. (2020). Cognitive behavioral therapy for menopausal symptoms. *Climacteric, 24*(1), 51–56. https://doi.org/10.1080/13697137.2020.1777965

Irish, L. A., Kline, C. E., Gunn, H. E., Buysse, D. J., & Hall, M. H. (2015). The role of sleep hygiene in promoting public health: A review of empirical evidence. *Sleep Medicine Reviews, 22,* 23–36. https://doi.org/10.1016/j.smrv.2014.10.001

Johnson, A., Roberts, L., & Elkins, G. (2019). Complementary and alternative medicine for menopause. *Journal of Evidence-Based Integrative Medicine, 24.* https://doi.org/10.1177/2515690X19829380

Kynaston, H. (2019). *Self-compassion: The secret of self-compassion: Learn self-compassion and self-love using tried-and-tested, proven methods.* Herman Kynaston.

Lillis, C., McNamara, M., Wheelan, J., McManus, M., Murphy, M. B., Lane, A., & Heavey P. M. (2021). *Experiences and health behaviours of menopausal women in Ireland.*

Lloyd, B., & Reed, M. (2018). *Health psychology.* Scientific e-Resources.

Mann, E., Smith, M. J., Hellier, J., Balabanovic, J. A., Hamed, H., Grunfeld, E. A., & Hunter, M. S. (2012). Cognitive behavioural treatment for women who have menopausal symptoms after breast cancer treatment (MENOS 1): A randomised controlled trial. *Lancet Oncology/Lancet Oncology, 13*(3), 309–318. https://doi.org/10.1016/s1470-2045(11)70364-3

Mariscal-de-Gante, Á., Palencia-Esteban, A., Grubanov-Boskovic, S., & Fernández-Macías, E. (2023). Feminization, ageing, and occupational change in Europe in the last 25 years. *Population and Development Review*, 49(4), 939–966. https://doi.org/10.1111/padr.12586

Masters, W. H., & Johnson, V. E. (1970). *Human sexual inadequacy*. Little Brown.

Mattern, S. (2021). *The slow moon climbs: The science, history, and meaning of menopause*. Princeton University Press.

McCall, D., & Potter, N. (2022). *Menopausing: The positive roadmap to your second spring*. HarperCollins UK.

Miguel, I., Von Humboldt, S., & Leal, I. (2024). Sexual well-being across the lifespan: Is sexual satisfaction related to adjustment to aging? *Sexuality Research and Social Policy*. https://doi.org/10.1007/s13178-024-00939-y

Morin, A. (2014). 7 scientifically proven benefits of gratitude that will motivate you to give thanks year-round. *Forbes.com*.

Mosconi, L. (2024). *The menopause brain: The new science empowering women to navigate midlife with knowledge and confidence*. Atlantic Books.

Muir, K. (2023). *Everything you need to know about the menopause (but were too afraid to ask)*. Gallery UK.

Myers, D. G. (2023). *How do we know ourselves? Curiosities and marvels of the human mind*. Picador USA.

Myers, D. G., & Spencer, S. J. (2006). *Social psychology*. McGraw-Hill Ryerson.

Newson, L. (2019). *Menopause: All you need to know in one concise manual: Signs and symptoms – time to rethink HRT – holistic treatments – coping at work – advice for all the family*. Haynes Publishing UK.

O'Donnell, A. T., & Habenicht, A. E. (2021). Stigma is associated with illness self-concept in individuals with concealable chronic illnesses. *British Journal of Health Psychology*, 27(1), 136–158. https://doi.org/10.1111/bjhp.12534

Ogden, J. (2019). *Health psychology* (6th ed.). McGraw Hill.

Pennington, D. C. (1986). *Essential social psychology*. Hodder Arnold.

Percival, M. (2023). *The psychology of counselling*. Taylor & Francis.

Rohleder, N. (2019). Stress and inflammation – the need to address the gap in the transition between acute and chronic stress effects. *Psychoneuroendocrinology*, 105, 164–171. https://doi.org/10.1016/j.psyneuen.2019.02.021

Robertson, G. (2020). *The ten steps of positive ageing: A handbook for personal change in later life*. Bloomsbury Publishing.

Rudnicka, E., Napierała, P., Podfigurna, A., Męczekalski, B., Smolarczyk, R., & Grymowicz, M. (2020). The World Health Organization (WHO) approach to healthy ageing. *Maturitas*, 139, 6–11. https://doi.org/10.1016/j.maturitas.2020.05.018

Rydberg, A., & Vegunata, S. (2023). *My body is beautiful: Sexual self-esteem and body esteem*. Retrieved October 2023, from https://mcpressmayoclinic.org

Shifren, J. L., & Gass, M. L. (2014). The North American menopause society recommendations for clinical care of midlife women. *Menopause the Journal of the North American Menopause Society*, 21(10), 1038–1062. https://doi.org/10.1097/gme.0000000000000319

Siegel, D. J. (2010). *The mindful therapist: A clinician's guide to mindsight and neural integration (Norton series on interpersonal neurobiology)*. W. W. Norton & Company.

Smith, K. (2014). Mental health: A world of depression. *Nature*, 515(7526), 180–181. https://doi.org/10.1038/515180a

Sohal, M., Singh, P., Dhillon, B. S., & Gill, H. S. (2022). Efficacy of journaling in the management of mental illness: A systematic review and meta-analysis. *Family Medicine and Community Health*, 10(1), e001154. https://doi.org/10.1136/fmch-2021-001154

Spence, S. H. (2013). *Psychosexual therapy: A cognitive-behavioural approach*. Springer.

Stanley, E. (2019). *Widen the window: Training your brain and body to thrive during stress and recover from trauma*. Hachette UK.

Steckenrider, J. (2023). Sexual activity of older adults: Let's talk about it. *The Lancet Healthy Longevity*, 4(3), e96–e97. https://doi.org/10.1016/s2666-7568(23)00003-x

Stevens, R. (1996). *Understanding the self*. SAGE.

Talaulikar, V. (2022). Menopause transition: Physiology and symptoms. *Baillière's Best Practice and Research in Clinical Obstetrics and Gynaecology*, 81, 3–7. https://doi.org/10.1016/j.bpobgyn.2022.03.003

Thomas, H. N., Chang, C. C. H., Dillon, S., & Hess, R. (2014). Sexual activity in midlife women: Importance of sex matters. *JAMA Internal Medicine*, 174(4), 631–633.

Vivian-Taylor, J., & Hickey, M. (2014). Menopause and depression: Is there a link? *Maturitas*, 79(2), 142–146. https://doi.org/10.1016/j.maturitas.2014.05.014

Von Hippel, C., Adhia, A., Rosenberg, S., Austin, S. B., Partridge, A., & Tamimi, R. (2019). Sexual function among women in midlife: Findings from the Nurses' Health Study II. *Women's Health Issues*, 29(4), 291–298. https://doi.org/10.1016/j.whi.2019.04.006

Vosper, J., Irons, C., Mackenzie-White, K., Saunders, F., Lewis, R., & Gibson, S. (2021). Introducing compassion focused psychosexual therapy. *Sexual & Relationship Therapy*, 38(3), 320–352. https://doi.org/10.1080/14681994.2021.1902495

Weber, M. T., Rubin, L. H., & Maki, P. M. (2013). Cognition in perimenopause. *Menopause the Journal of the North American Menopause Society*, *20*(5), 511–517. https://doi.org/10.1097/gme.0b013e31827655e5

Williams, F. (2017). *The nature fix: Why nature makes us happier, healthier, and more creative.* W. W. Norton & Company.

Wilson, R. A. (1966). *Feminine forever.* M. Evans.

Wood, W., & Rünger, D. (2016). Psychology of habit. *Annual Review of Psychology*, *67*(1), 289–314. https://doi.org/10.1146/annurev-psych-122414-033417

Wright et al. cited in The Oxford Handbook of Stress and Mental Health. (2018). *eBooks.* Oxford University Press. https://doi.org/10.1093/oxfordhb/9780190681777.001.0001

Zeanah, P. D., & Schwarz, J. C. (1996). Reliability and validity of the sexual self-esteem inventory for women. *Assessment*, *3*(1), 1–15. https://doi.org/10.1177/107319119600300101

FURTHER READING AND WEB RESOURCES

The following are useful resources on topics presented in each chapter.

CHAPTER 1 – MENOPAUSE THROUGH THE AGES

BOOKS

Avis, N. E., Crawford, S. L., & Green, R. (2018). Vasomotor symptoms across the menopause transition. *Obstetrics and Gynecology Clinics of North America*, 45(4), 629–640. https://doi.org/10.1016/j.ogc.2018.07.005

Bezzant, N. (2022). *This changes everything: The honest guide to menopause and perimenopause.* Penguin Books.

Foxcroft, L. (2010). *Hot flushes, cold science: A history of the modern menopause.* Granta Books.

Hunter, M., & Smith, M. (2024). *Living well through the menopause: An evidence-based cognitive behavioural guide.* Hachette UK.

McCall, D., & Potter, N. (2022). *Menopausing: The positive roadmap to your second spring.* HarperCollins UK.

WEBSITES

British Menopause Society. www.thebms.org.uk

North American Menopause Society. www.menopause.org

The Menopause Hub, www.themenopuasehub.ie

CHAPTER 2 – UNDERSTANDING AND MANAGING MENOPAUSE – HOW CAN PSYCHOLOGY HELP?

BOOKS

Albery, I., & Munafo, M. (2008). *Key concepts in health psychology*. SAGE.

Jarrett, C. (2011). *30-second psychology: The 50 most thought-provoking psychology theories, each explained in half a minute*. Icon Books Ltd.

WEBSITES

APA Handbook of Health Psychology. www.apa.org-health-psychology

The Psychology of Menopause. www.thepsychologyofmenopause.com

CHAPTER 3 – PSYCHOLOGICAL HEALTH AND BRAIN HEALTH

BOOKS

Antonovsky, A. (2002). Unravelling the mystery of health: How people manage stress and stay well. In *eBooks* (pp. 127–139). SAGE Publications Ltd. https://doi.org/10.4135/9781446221129.n9

Baglioni, C., Espie, C. A., & Riemann, D. (2022). *Cognitive-behavioural therapy for insomnia (CBT-I) across the life span: Guidelines and clinical protocols for health professionals*. John Wiley & Sons.

Gillihan, S. J. (2020). *Cognitive behavioural therapy made simple: 10 strategies for managing anxiety, depression, anger, panic and worry*. Hachette UK.

Marsico, K. (2013). *Depression and stress*. Cavendish Square Publishing, LLC.

Mosconi, L. (2024). *The menopause brain: The new science empowering women to navigate midlife with knowledge and confidence*. Atlantic Books.

Percival, M. (2023). *The psychology of counselling*. Taylor & Francis.

Saboowala, H. K. (2022). *What is brain fog? Symptoms, causes & treatment*. Dr. Hakim Saboowala.

Shaffer, A. (2020). *How to beat stress: The scientific guide to being happy*. Centennial Books.

WEBSITES

Healthy Brains by Cleveland Clinic. www.healthybrains.org

MP Psychological Services. www.mppsychologicalservices.com

CHAPTER 4 – THE SELF IN TRANSITION

BOOKS

Myers, D. G. (2023). *How do we know ourselves? Curiosities and marvels of the human mind.* Picador USA.

Vargas, R. (2016). *Body image: Social influences, ethnic differences and impact on self-esteem.* Nova Science Publishers.

CHAPTER 5 – SEXUAL WELL-BEING DURING AND AFTER MENOPAUSE

BOOKS

Shub, J., & Allena, G. (2019). *Sex positive now: Everything you need to know about sex positivity.* Jeremy Shub Counselling.

Weiner, L., & Avery-Clark, C. (2017). *Sensate focus in sex therapy: The illustrated manual.* Routledge.

WEBSITES

Sex Therapist St. Louis. www.sextherapistsstlouis.com

CHAPTER 6 – A LIFE WORTH LIVING - POSITIVE PSYCHOLOGY AND POSITIVE AGEING

BOOKS

Harris, R. (2013). *The happiness trap: Stop struggling, start living.* Exisle Publishing.

Papek, S. (2022). *Age is your edge: How to find purpose and fulfilment in midlife.* BookLocker. com, Inc.

Seligman, M. (2011). *Authentic happiness: Using the new positive psychology to realise your potential for lasting fulfilment.* Hachette UK.

Seligman, M. (2018). *Learned optimism: How to change your mind and your life.* Hachette UK.

WEBSITES

Age UK. www.ageuk.org.uk

Centre for Ageing Better. www.ageing-better.org.uk

Live Better, Longer. www.bluezones.com

CHAPTER 7 – ESTABLISHING AND MAINTAINING WELLNESS DURING AND AFTER MENOPAUSE

Braime, H. (2016). *From coping to thriving: How to turn self-care into a way of life.* Hannah Braime.

Clear, J. (2018). *Atomic habits: An easy & proven way to build good habits & break bad ones.* https:// catalog.umj.ac.id/index.php?p=show_detail&id=62390

Cocca-Leffler, M. (2021). *The power of yet.* Abrams.

James, B. (2021). *Secrets to getting good sleep: Tips, sleep hygiene & how to fight sleep insomnia.* Abbott Properties.

Kynaston, H. (2019). *Self-compassion: The secret of self-compassion: Learn self-compassion and self-love using tried-and-tested, proven methods.*

Noonan, S. J. (2013). *Managing your depression: What you can do to feel better.* JHU Press.

Passy, C. (2021). *Surprising benefits of journaling: Superpowers to take over the world: How to increase productivity.*

Sciandra, K. (2015). *The mindfulness habit: Six weeks to creating the habit of being present.* Llewellyn Worldwide.

Williams, F. (2017). *The nature fix: Why nature makes us happier, healthier, and more creative.* W. W. Norton & Company.

WEBSITES

Positive Psychology Center – University of Pennsylvania. www.ppc.sas.upenn.edu

Printed in the United States
by Baker & Taylor Publisher Services